Lesbian, Gay, Bisexual, and Transgender Youth

Editors

STEWART L. ADELSON
NADIA L. DOWSHEN
HARVEY J. MAKADON
ROBERT GAROFALO

PEDIATRIC CLINICS
OF NORTH AMERICA

www.pediatric.theclinics.com

Consulting Editor
BONITA F. STANTON

December 2016 • Volume 63 • Number 6

ELSEVIER

1600 John F. Kennedy Boulevard • Suite 1800 • Philadelphia, Pennsylvania, 19103-2899

http://www.theclinics.com

THE PEDIATRIC CLINICS OF NORTH AMERICA Volume 63, Number 6
December 2016 ISSN 0031-3955, ISBN-13: 978-0-323-47747-5

Editor: Kerry Holland
Developmental Editor: Casey Jackson

The Pediatric Clinics of North America (ISSN 0031-3955) is published bimonthly by Elsevier Inc., 360 Park Avenue South, New York, NY 10010-1710. Months of issue are February, April, June, August, October, and December. Periodicals postage paid at New York, NY and additional mailing offices. Subscription prices are $200.00 per year (US individuals), $556.00 per year (US institutions), $270.00 per year (Canadian individuals), $740.00 per year (Canadian institutions), $325.00 per year (international individuals), $740.00 per year (international institutions), $100.00 per year (US students and residents), and $165.00 per year (international and Canadian residents and students). To receive students/resident rare, orders must be accompanied by name of affiliated institution, date of term, and the signature of program/residency coordinator on institution letterhead. Orders will be billed at individual rate until proof of status is received. Foreign air speed delivery is included in all *Clinics* subscription prices. All prices are subject to change without notice. **POSTMASTER:** Send address changes to *The Pediatric Clinics of North America*, Elsevier Health Sciences Division, Subscription Customer Service, 3251 Riverport Lane, Maryland Heights, MO 63043. **Customer Service: 1-800-654-2452 (US and Canada). From outside of the US and Canada: 1-314-447-8871. Fax: 1-314-447-8029. For print support, E-mail: JournalsCustomerService-usa@elsevier.com. For online support, E-mail: JournalsOnlineSupport-usa@elsevier.com.**

Reprints. For copies of 100 or more, of articles in this publication, please contact the Commercial Reprints Department, Elsevier Inc., 360 Park Avenue South, New York, NY 10010-1710. Tel.: 212-633-3874; Fax: 212-633-3820; E-mail: reprints@elsevier.com.

The Pediatric Clinics of North America is also published in Spanish by McGraw-Hill Inter-americana Editores S.A., Mexico City, Mexico; in Portuguese by Riechmann and Affonso Editores, Rua Comandante Coelho 1085, CEP 21250, Rio de Janeiro, Brazil; and in Greek by Althayia SA, Athens, Greece.

The Pediatric Clinics of North America is covered in *MEDLINE/PubMed (Index Medicus)*, *Excerpta Medica*, *Current Contents*, *Current Contents/Clinical Medicine*, *Science Citation Index*, *ASCA*, *ISI/BIOMED*, and *BIOSIS*.

PROGRAM OBJECTIVE
The goal of the *Pediatric Clinics of North America* is to keep practicing physicians and residents up to date with current clinical practice in pediatrics by providing timely articles reviewing the state-of-the-art in patient care.

TARGET AUDIENCE
All practicing pediatricians, physicians and healthcare professionals who provide patient care to pediatric patients.

LEARNING OBJECTIVES
Upon completion of this activity, participants will be able to:
1. Review topics including bullying, minority stress, family acceptance, and mental health for lesbian, gay, bisexual, and transgender (LGBT) youth.
2. Discuss issues in sexual health for LGBT youth.
3. Recognize sociocultural factors, including affirmative environments and family dynamics, in development and mental health of LGBT youth.

ACCREDITATION
The Elsevier Office of Continuing Medical Education (EOCME) is accredited by the Accreditation Council for Continuing Medical Education (ACCME) to provide continuing medical education for physicians.

The EOCME designates this enduring material for a maximum of 15 *AMA PRA Category 1 Credit*(s)™. Physicians should claim only the credit commensurate with the extent of their participation in the activity.

All other health care professionals requesting continuing education credit for this enduring material will be issued a certificate of participation.

DISCLOSURE OF CONFLICTS OF INTEREST
The EOCME assesses conflict of interest with its instructors, faculty, planners, and other individuals who are in a position to control the content of CME activities. All relevant conflicts of interest that are identified are thoroughly vetted by EOCME for fair balance, scientific objectivity, and patient care recommendations. EOCME is committed to providing its learners with CME activities that promote improvements or quality in healthcare and not a specific proprietary business or a commercial interest.

The planning committee, staff, authors and editors listed below have identified no financial relationships or relationships to products or devices they or their spouse/life partner have with commercial interest related to the content of this CME activity:
Stewart L. Adelson, MD; Romulo Alcalde Aromin Jr, MD, FAPA; Laura M. Bogart, PhD; Peggy T. Cohen-Kettenis, PhD; Annelou L.C. de Vries, MD, PhD; Nadia Dowshen, MD; Valerie A. Earnshaw, PhD; Anjali Fortna; Scott E. Hadland, MD, MPH, MS; Mark L. Hatzenbuehler, PhD; Kerry Holland; Sabra L. Katz-Wise, PhD; Daniel Klink, MD, PhD; Indu Kumari; Harvey J. Makadon, MD, FACP; Zachary McClain, MD; Anthony Morgan, AAS; Warren Ng, MD; John E. Pachankis, PhD; Rebecka Peebles, MD; V. Paul Poteat, PhD; Sari L. Reisner, ScD; Margaret Rosario, PhD; Caroline Salas-Humara, MD; Renata Arrington Sanders, MD, MPH, ScM; Mark A. Schuster, MD, PhD; Bonita F. Stanton, MD; Megan Suermann; Oliver M. Stroeh, MD; Cynthia J. Telingator, MD; Michael Tsappis, MD; Cecil R. Webster Jr, MD; Sarah M. Wood, MD; Baligh R. Yehia, MD, MPP, MSc.

The planning committee, staff, authors and editors listed below have identified financial relationships or relationships to products or devices they or their spouse/life partner have with commercial interest related to the content of this CME activity:
Errol Fields, MD, PhD, MPH is a consultant/advisor for Gilead.
Robert Garofalo, MD, MPH is a consultant/advisor for Gilead.

UNAPPROVED/OFF-LABEL USE DISCLOSURE
The EOCME requires CME faculty to disclose to the participants:
1. When products or procedures being discussed are off-label, unlabelled, experimental, and/or investigational (not US Food and Drug Administration [FDA] approved); and
2. Any limitations on the information presented, such as data that are preliminary or that represent ongoing research, interim analyses, and/or unsupported opinions. Faculty may discuss information about pharmaceutical agents that is outside of FDA-approved labelling. This information is intended solely for CME

and is not intended to promote off-label use of these medications. If you have any questions, contact the medical affairs department of the manufacturer for the most recent prescribing information.

TO ENROLL

To enroll in the *Pediatric Clinics of North America* Continuing Medical Education program, call customer service at 1-800-654-2452 or sign up online at http://www.theclinics.com/home/cme. The CME program is available to subscribers for an additional annual fee of USD 290.

METHOD OF PARTICIPATION

In order to claim credit, participants must complete the following:
1. Complete enrolment as indicated above.
2. Read the activity.
3. Complete the CME Test and Evaluation. Participants must achieve a score of 70% on the test. All CME Tests and Evaluations must be completed online.

CME INQUIRIES/SPECIAL NEEDS

For all CME inquiries or special needs, please contact elsevierCME@elsevier.com.

Contributors

CONSULTING EDITOR

BONITA F. STANTON, MD
Founding Dean, School of Medicine, Professor of Pediatrics, Seton Hall University, South Orange, New Jersey

EDITORS

STEWART L. ADELSON, MD
Assistant Clinical Professor, Department of Psychiatry, Columbia University College of Physicians and Surgeons; Adjunct Clinical Assistant Professor, Department of Psychiatry, Weill Cornell Medical College, New York, New York

NADIA L. DOWSHEN, MD
Director of Adolescent HIV Services, Co-Director, Gender and Sexuality Development Clinic, Craig-Dalsimer Division of Adolescent Medicine, Faculty, PolicyLab, Children's Hospital of Philadelphia, Assistant Professor of Pediatrics, Perelman School of Medicine, University of Pennsylvania, Philadelphia, Pennsylvania

HARVEY J. MAKADON, MD, FACP
Director of Education and Training Programs, The Fenway Institute, Professor of Medicine, Harvard Medical School, Boston, Massachusetts

ROBERT GAROFALO, MD, MPH
Division Chief, Adolescent Medicine, Director, Center for Gender, Sexuality and HIV Prevention, Ann & Robert H. Lurie Children's Hospital of Chicago, Professor of Pediatrics and Preventive Medicine, Northwestern University Feinberg School of Medicine, Chicago, Illinois

AUTHORS

STEWART L. ADELSON, MD
Assistant Clinical Professor, Department of Psychiatry, Columbia University College of Physicians and Surgeons; Adjunct Clinical Assistant Professor, Department of Psychiatry, Weill Cornell Medical College, New York, New York

ROMULO ALCALDE AROMIN Jr, MD, FAPA
Associate Director, Psychiatry, Psychosocial Services, Institute for Family Health, New York, New York

LAURA M. BOGART, PhD
Research Director, Division of General Pediatrics, Boston Children's Hospital; Associate Professor, Department of Pediatrics, Harvard Medical School; Senior Behavioral Scientist, Health Unit, RAND Corporation, Santa Monica, California

PEGGY T. COHEN-KETTENIS, PhD
Professor Emeritus of Medical Psychology, Department of Medical Psychology,
VU University Medical Center, Amsterdam, The Netherlands

ANNELOU L.C. DE VRIES, MD, PhD
Child and Adolescent Psychiatrist, Department of Child and Adolescent Psychiatry,
VU University Medical Center, Amsterdam, The Netherlands

NADIA L. DOWSHEN, MD
Director of Adolescent HIV Services, Co-Director, Gender and Sexuality Development
Clinic, Craig-Dalsimer Division of Adolescent Medicine, Faculty, PolicyLab, Children's
Hospital of Philadelphia, Assistant Professor of Pediatrics, Perelman School of Medicine,
University of Pennsylvania, Philadelphia, Pennsylvania

VALERIE A. EARNSHAW, PhD
Associate Scientific Researcher, Division of General Pediatrics, Boston Children's
Hospital; Instructor, Department of Pediatrics, Harvard Medical School, Boston,
Massachusetts

ERROL FIELDS, MD, PhD, MPH
Assistant Professor of Pediatrics, Division of General Pediatrics and Adolescent
Medicine, Johns Hopkins School of Medicine, Baltimore, Maryland

SCOTT E. HADLAND, MD, MPH, MS
Instructor, Division of Adolescent/Young Adult Medicine, Department of Medicine,
Boston Children's Hospital; Department of Pediatrics, Harvard Medical School, Boston,
Massachusetts

MARK L. HATZENBUEHLER, PhD
Associate Professor, Department of Sociomedical Sciences, Mailman School of Public
Health, Columbia University, New York, New York

SABRA L. KATZ-WISE, PhD
Research Scientist, Division of Adolescent/Young Adult Medicine, Boston Children's
Hospital; Instructor, Department of Pediatrics, Harvard Medical School, Boston,
Massachusetts

DANIEL KLINK, MD, PhD
Pediatric Endocrinologist, Division of Endocrinology, Department of Pediatrics,
VU University Medical Center, Amsterdam, The Netherlands

HARVEY J. MAKADON, MD, FACP
Director of Education and Training Programs, The Fenway Institute, Professor of
Medicine, Harvard Medical School, Boston, Massachusetts

ZACHARY McCLAIN, MD
Assistant Professor of Pediatrics, Perelman School of Medicine, University of
Pennsylvania; Craig Dalsimer Division of Adolescent Medicine, The Children's Hospital of
Philadelphia, Philadelphia, Pennsylvania

ANTHONY MORGAN, AAS
Research Program Coordinator, Division of General Pediatrics and Adolescent Medicine,
Johns Hopkins School of Medicine, Baltimore, Maryland

YIU KEE WARREN NG, MD
Associate Professor of Psychiatry, Division of Child & Adolescent Psychiatry, Columbia University College of Physicians & Surgeons, New York, New York

JOHN E. PACHANKIS, PhD
Associate Professor of Epidemiology (Chronic Diseases), Yale School of Public Health, New Haven, Connecticut

REBECKA PEEBLES, MD
Assistant Professor of Pediatrics, Perelman School of Medicine, University of Pennsylvania; Craig Dalsimer Division of Adolescent Medicine, The Children's Hospital of Philadelphia, Philadelphia, Pennsylvania

V. PAUL POTEAT, PhD
Associate Professor, Counseling, Developmental, and Educational Psychology Department, Boston College, Chestnut Hill, Massachusetts

SARI L. REISNER, ScD
Associate Scientific Researcher, Division of General Pediatrics, Boston Children's Hospital; Assistant Professor, Department of Pediatrics, Harvard Medical School; Assistant Professor, Department of Epidemiology, Harvard T.H. Chan School of Public Health; Affiliated Research Scientist, The Fenway Institute, Boston, Massachusetts

MARGARET ROSARIO, PhD
Professor, Department of Psychology, City University of New York–City College and Graduate Center, New York, New York

CAROLINE SALAS-HUMARA, MD
Assistant Professor, Department of Pediatrics and Adolescent Medicine, NYU School of Medicine, New York, New York

RENATA ARRINGTON SANDERS, MD, MPH, ScM
Assistant Professor, Division of General Pediatrics and Adolescent Medicine, Johns Hopkins School of Medicine, Baltimore, Maryland

MARK A. SCHUSTER, MD, PhD
Chief, Division of General Pediatrics, Boston Children's Hospital; William Berenberg Professor, Department of Pediatrics, Harvard Medical School, Boston, Massachusetts

OLIVER M. STROEH, MD
Clarice Kestenbaum, MD Assistant Professor of Education and Training, Division of Child & Adolescent Psychiatry, Columbia University College of Physicians & Surgeons, New York, New York

CYNTHIA J. TELINGATOR, MD
Assistant Professor in Psychiatry, Division of Child and Adolescent Psychiatry, Cambridge Health Alliance, Harvard Medical School, Cambridge, Massachusetts

MICHAEL TSAPPIS, MD
Associate, Divisions of Adolescent Medicine and Psychiatry, Boston Children's Hospital; Instructor, Department of Psychiatry, Harvard Medical School, Boston, Massachusetts

CECIL R. WEBSTER Jr, MD
Instructor in Psychiatry, Part-Time, Division of Child and Adolescent Psychiatry, Cambridge Health Alliance, Harvard Medical School, Cambridge, Massachusetts

SARAH M. WOOD, MD
Adolescent Medicine Fellow, Craig-Dalsimer Division of Adolescent Medicine, Children's Hospital of Philadelphia; Instructor, Department of Pediatrics, University of Pennsylvania School of Medicine, Philadelphia, Pennsylvania

BALIGH R. YEHIA, MD, MPP, MSc
Adjunct Assistant Professor of Medicine, Department of Medicine; Penn Medicine Program for LGBT Health, Perelman School of Medicine, University of Pennsylvania, Philadelphia, Pennsylvania

Contents

> Lesbian, gay, bisexual, transgender, queer and questioning (LGBTQ) youth
> may experience interpersonal and structural stigma within the health care
> environment. This article begins by reviewing special considerations for
> the care of LGBTQ youth, then turns to systems-level principles underlying
> inclusive and affirming care. It then examines specific strategies that indi-
> vidual providers can use to provide more patient-centered care, and con-
> cludes with a discussion of how clinics and health systems can tailor
> clinical services to the needs of LGBTQ youth.

> Assessing, monitoring, and supporting children and adolescents' mental
> health are integral parts of comprehensive pediatric primary care. These
> are especially relevant for LGBT youth, who frequently experience unique
> stressors, often including having an identity different from family and peer
> expectations, whether to reveal it, and stigma like peer bullying, family
> rejection, social intolerance, and self nonacceptance. Pediatricians should
> know key mental health practice principles for LGBT youth, how to adapt
> these to various pediatric settings, the continuum of mental health inter-
> ventions, and their local resources. Practice principles in pediatric care
> for LGBT youth and examples of their implementation are discussed.

> In this article, we review theory and evidence on stigma and minority stress
> as social/structural determinants of health among lesbian, gay, bisexual,
> and transgender (LGBT) youth. We discuss different forms of stigma at in-
> dividual (eg, identity concealment), interpersonal (eg, victimization), and
> structural (eg, laws and social norms) levels, as well as the mechanisms

linking stigma to adverse health outcomes among LGBT youth. Finally, we discuss clinical (eg, cognitive behavioral therapy) and public health (eg, antibullying policies) interventions that effectively target stigma-inducing mechanisms to improve the health of LGBT youth.

Bullying of lesbian, gay, bisexual, and transgender (LGBT) youth is prevalent in the United States, and represents LGBT stigma when tied to sexual orientation and/or gender identity or expression. LGBT youth commonly report verbal, relational, and physical bullying, and damage to property. Bullying undermines the well-being of LGBT youth, with implications for risky health behaviors, poor mental health, and poor physical health that may last into adulthood. Pediatricians can play a vital role in preventing and identifying bullying, providing counseling to youth and their parents, and advocating for programs and policies to address LGBT bullying.

In this article, we address theories of attachment and parental acceptance and rejection, and their implications for lesbian, gay, bisexual, and transgender (LGBT) youths' identity and health. We also provide 2 clinical cases to illustrate the process of family acceptance of a transgender youth and a gender nonconforming youth who was neither a sexual minority nor transgender. Clinical implications of family acceptance and rejection of LGBT youth are discussed.

Lesbian, gay, bisexual, transgender (LGBT), and questioning youth represent a diverse population who are affected by many sexual health inequities, including increased risk for human immunodeficiency virus (HIV) and sexually transmitted infections (STIs). To provide comprehensive sexual health care for LGBT youth, providers should set the stage with a nonjudgmental, respectful tone. Providers should be competent in recognizing symptoms of STIs and HIV and aware of the most up-to-date screening guidelines for LGBT youth. Sexual health visits should also focus on prevention, including safer sex practices, HIV pre-exposure and post-exposure prophylaxis, family planning, and immunization for hepatitis and human papillomavirus.

Knowing how to manage substance abuse in all youth is an important aspect of pediatric care, including providing clinically appropriate anticipatory guidance, monitoring, assessment, and treatment. Although most lesbian, gay, bisexual, and transgender (LGBT) youth do not abuse substances, as a group they experience unique challenges in self-identity development that put them at an increased risk for substance abuse. This article addresses prevention and management of substance use in LGBT youth relevant to pediatrics and allied professions as an aspect of their overall health care. It reviews basic information about substance abuse in youth and special considerations for LGBT youth.

Adolescence is a crucial period for emerging sexual orientation and gender identity and also body image disturbance and disordered eating. Body image distortion and disordered eating are important pediatric problems affecting individuals along the sexual orientation and gender identity spectrum. Lesbian, gay, bisexual, transgender (LGBT) youth are at risk for eating disorders and body dissatisfaction. Disordered eating in LGBT and gender variant youth may be associated with poorer quality of life and mental health outcomes. Pediatricians should know that these problems occur more frequently in LGBT youth. There is evidence that newer treatment paradigms involving family support are more effective than individual models of care.

Intersectionality suggests that multiple social identities intersect at the individual or micro level of experience and reflects larger social structural inequities experienced on the macro level. This article uses intersectionality to describe how multiple stigmatized social identities can create unique challenges for young black gay and bisexual men (YBGBM). YBGBM exist at the intersection of multiple stigmatized identities compared with their majority peers. This article examines key intersecting identities and cultural expectations that exist in YBGBM and how those factors may predispose young men to adverse health outcomes and health inequality.

Families headed by sexual minorities encounter unique barriers to care and health equity despite greater cultural acceptance and visibility. Empirical research suggests that children in lesbian, gay, bisexual, and transgender (LGBT) families develop and function comparably to those from traditional families. In helping families, awareness of family structure is important. The health care provider should be familiar with family composition, and their community, social supports, race/ethnic concerns, financial issues, and other vulnerabilities. Cultivating an office culture and practice that supports all patients to comfortably discuss their family history, interpersonal experiences, needs, and vulnerabilities is essential for excellence in clinical care.

What the Primary Care Pediatrician Needs to Know About Gender Incongruence and Gender Dysphoria in Children and Adolescents   1121

Annelou L.C. de Vries, Daniel Klink, and Peggy T. Cohen-Kettenis

The recognition and acknowledgment that gender identity and birth-assigned sex may be incongruent in children and adolescents have evolved in recent decades. Transgender care for children and adolescents has developed and is now more widely available. Controversies exist, however, around clinical management of gender dysphoria and gender incongruence in children and adolescents. Clinical guidelines are consensus based and research evidence is limited. Puberty suppression as part of clinical management has become a valuable element of adolescent transgender care, but long-term evidence of success is limited. These uncertainties should be weighed against the risk of harming a transgender adolescent when medical intervention is denied.

PEDIATRIC CLINICS OF NORTH AMERICA

ISSUE OF RELATED INTEREST

Primary Care: Clinics in Office Practice, September 2014 (Vol. 41, Issue 3)
Adolescent Medicine
William B. Shore, Francesco Leanza, and Nicole Chaisson, *Editors*
www.primarycare.theclinics.com

THE CLINICS ARE AVAILABLE ONLINE!
Access your subscription at:
www.theclinics.com

Foreword

Lesbian, Gay, Bisexual, and Transgender Youth

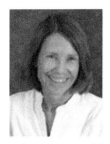

Bonita F. Stanton, MD
Consulting Editor

The preadolescent and adolescent periods are difficult for many—perhaps most—youth. Adolescents face a variety of changes, physical, physiologic, psychological, and environmental, all of which they must learn to navigate. Lesbian, gay, bisexual, and transgender (LGBT) youth face the traditional trials of adolescence, but in addition, a wide range of challenges, greatly influenced by the societies, communities, and families in which they reside and interact. Moreover, once thought to occur most commonly during adolescence, it now appears that on average self-recognition of LGBT orientation occurs prior to age 10.[1] Therefore, it is critically important for all pediatricians and child–health care providers, not just adolescent providers, to be knowledgeable about and comfortable in talking with LGBT children and youth to assist them in confronting the challenges and opportunities they may encounter, whether a function of growth and development or of their LGBT orientation.

Moreover, for a range of reasons, LGBT youth may face a higher likelihood of certain diseases and/or adverse social situations. For example, as most pediatricians are doubtless aware, LGBT face higher rates of several sexually transmitted diseases. In 2014, gay and bisexual men accounted for an estimated 83% (29,418) of HIV diagnoses among men and 67% of all diagnoses.[2] As another example, LGBT are much more likely to be homeless; while overall 5% to 10% of adolescents and young adults in the United States are LGBT, an estimated 20% to 40% of homeless adolescents are LGBT.[1]

Equally important, but perhaps less recognized by pediatricians, are structural inequalities resulting in stigma, facing LGBT, such as accommodations based on physical evidence of gender rather than sexual orientation. A parent, teacher, or physician unaware of the magnitude associated with such rules may unwittingly further complicate an already distressed youth.[3]

Pediatric practice requires a skillful mix of risk reduction and strength maximization. Effectively offering such counsel in the absence of a robust understanding of the hopes

http://dx.doi.org/10.1016/j.pcl.2016.09.003
0031-3955/16/© 2016 Published by Elsevier Inc.

and dreams, the fears and trials, the potential risks, and the available supports impacting LGBT children and youth is not possible.

This sensitively and thoughtfully organized and written description of the many aspects of sexual orientation and identity and their impact on childhood and adolescence is a must-read for all child–health care providers. I suspect that there is no one who reads this who will not learn from it—and in so doing, become a better pediatrician and/or child–health care provider. Through such enhanced understanding, we can help to normalize what is not a sickness or disability but just a variation within normal maturation and development.

Bonita F. Stanton, MD
School of Medicine
Seton Hall University
400 South Orange Avenue
South Orange, NJ 07079, USA

E-mail address:
bonita.stanton@shu.edu

REFERENCES

1. Center for American Progress. Gay and Transgender Youth Homelessness by the Numbers. Available at: https://www.americanprogress.org/issues/lgbt/news/2010/06/21/7980/gay-and-transgender-youth-homelessness-by-the-numbers/.
2. Centers for Disease Control and Prevention. HIV in the United States: At A Glance. Available at: http://www.cdc.gov/hiv/statistics/overview/ataglance.html.
3. Meyer IH. Prejudice, social stress, and mental health in lesbian, gay, and bisexual populations: conceptual issues and research evidence. Psych Bull 2003;129(5): 674–97.

Preface

Introduction to Lesbian, Gay, Bisexual, and Transgender Youth Health

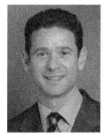

Stewart L. Adelson, MD

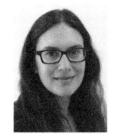

Nadia L. Dowshen, MD

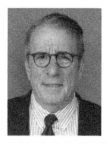

Harvey J Makadon, MD, FACP

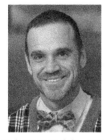

Robert Garofalo, MD,
MPH

Editors

In recent years, the pediatric literature and leading organizations including the American Academy of Pediatrics, the Institute of Medicine, the American Academy of Child and Adolescent Psychiatry, and the World Professional Association of Transgender Health have drawn attention to the pressing physical and mental health needs of lesbian, gay, bisexual, and transgender (LGBT) youth.[1–4] This issue is intended to help clinical practitioners of pediatrics and allied professions to understand and respond to these needs. In doing so, it addresses health care not only of youth who already identify themselves or are perceived by others as LGBT but also of those who might be on developmental paths that include these.

Nonheterosexual orientations and nonconformity in gender expression are not uncommon in youth, and part of normal development. However, in addition to the normal health and mental health needs they share with all youth, certain aspects of LGBT youths' development are unique. As LGBT youth are becoming increasingly visible

Pediatr Clin N Am 63 (2016) xvii–xxi
http://dx.doi.org/10.1016/j.pcl.2016.09.002
0031-3955/16/© 2016 Published by Elsevier Inc.

pediatric.theclinics.com

in society, competence in caring for them and families is a core skill that is necessary for all pediatric practitioners.

This issue is framed around key concepts. These include the *biopsychosocial model*, in which mental and physical health are interconnected and related to social factors, sexuality, and gender during development. There is *epidemiologic evidence* of special health needs among the pediatric LGBT population, including increased *risk* for certain illnesses associated with significant morbidity and mortality. In part, this is because LGBT youth are exposed to certain *epidemics* affecting them, including HIV, and certain substances of abuse. A substantial body of evidence indicates that risk is mediated by others' reactions to LGBT youth, including *stigma* that may adversely affect their physical and mental health in a variety of ways. This includes both interpersonal stigma, such as family, peer bullying, violence, or other forms of interpersonal discrimination, and also structural stigma, which may affect equity in health care resources, training, and competence. The concept that stigma mediates adverse health outcomes is known as the *minority stress model*.[5] The framework of *intersectionality* described in this issue refers to the way in which sociocultural factors in addition to LGBT-specific ones, including race/ethnicity, related stigma, and economic factors, can interact to influence health.

Although they are exposed to unique risks, LGBT youth also display patterns of strength and *resilience* that mitigate the likelihood of adverse outcomes. In each youth, a personal profile of vulnerability and strength influences how the individual copes with stressors and other risk exposure. Good clinical practice includes not only addressing risk but also enhancing strength to promote adaptive coping, good physical and mental health, and optimal fulfillment of each youth's developmental potential.

Clinical practitioners of pediatrics and allied professions have opportunities to promote health and well-being in LGBT youth through a variety of recognized medical interventions ranging from anticipatory guidance to specialized care. These include supporting healthy emotional development and providing comprehensive, inclusive sexual health education, addressing special needs like HIV prevention and treatment and, for transgender youth, appropriately providing gender-affirming care. This issue discusses clinical competence in these and other areas of physical and mental health for LGBT youth.

An increasing evidence base guides best pediatric practice with LGBT youth. This issue refers to that evidence and expert guidelines wherever available. Several articles also point to gaps in the literature where more research is needed. In light of these gaps, clinicians must sometimes generalize limited evidence derived from research settings and existing practice guidelines to novel contexts in primary care and other community settings. Therefore, in addition to using best practice guidelines whenever possible, this issue discusses using informed consent principles when it is not. Where there are controversies about best practice, this issue discusses them transparently. As this series is geared toward those caring for children and adolescents in clinical practice, there is a pragmatic focus on the clinical application of knowledge in the context of community, family, and development, with illustrative case vignettes.

At present, significant barriers exist to addressing the physical and mental health needs of LGBT youth and contribute to significant health inequities in this population. This issue is intended as a tool to help practitioners of pediatrics and allied professions to provide improved care, research, and education to meet these needs.

DEFINITIONS

As knowledge about caring for LGBT youth grows, concepts and terminology evolve. This issue explicitly defines key current terms for clarity, recognizing that their semantics are to a certain degree arbitrary and that other definitions are in use or may emerge in the future. The following terms are reprinted from the American Academy of Child and Adolescent Psychiatry's Practice Parameter on LGBT youth and are referred to throughout the issue.

AMERICAN ACADEMY OF CHILD AND ADOLESCENT PSYCHIATRY LESBIAN, GAY, BISEXUAL, AND TRANSGENDER YOUTH PRACTICE PARAMETER DEFINITIONS

- *Sex*, in the sense of being male or female, refers to a person's anatomical sex. (Although usually considered dichotomously male or female, disorders of sex development can lead to intersex conditions, which are beyond the scope of this practice parameter.)
- *Gender* refers to the perception of a person's sex on the part of society as male or female.
- *Gender role behavior* refers to activities, interests, use of symbols, styles, or other personal and social attributes that are recognized as masculine or feminine.
- *Gender identity* refers to an individual's personal sense of self as male or female. It usually develops by age 3, is concordant with a person's sex and gender, and remains stable over the lifetime. For a small number of individuals, it can change later in life. For some individuals, gender identity differs from sex assigned at birth. In others it may be non-binary – that is, not able to be categorized as just male or female; it may be both, neither, or another gender.
- *Identity* refers to one's abstract sense of self within a cultural and social matrix. This broader meaning (equivalent to ego identity) is distinct from gender identity and is usually consolidated in adolescence.
- *Sexual orientation* refers to the sex of the person to whom an individual is erotically attracted. It comprises several components, including sexual fantasy, patterns of physiologic arousal, sexual behavior, sexual identity, and social role.
  - ○ *Homosexual* people are attracted erotically to people of the same sex and are commonly referred to as gay in the case of males, and gay or lesbian in the case of females.
  - ○ *Heterosexual* people are attracted erotically to people of the other sex.
  - ○ *Bisexual* people are attracted erotically to people of both sexes.
- *Sexual minority* refers to homosexual and bisexual youth and adults.
- *Sexual prejudice* (or more archaically, **homophobia**) refers to bias against homosexual people. "Homophobia" is technically not a phobia; like other prejudices, it is characterized by hostility and is thus a misnomer, but the term is used colloquially.[6]
- *Internalized Sexual Prejudice* (or colloquially, *"**Internalizd Homophobia**"*) is a syndrome of self-loathing based upon the adoption of anti-homosexual attitudes by homosexual people themselves.
- *Heterosexism* refers to individual and societal assumptions—sometimes not explicitly recognized—promoting heterosexuality to the disadvantage of other sexual orientations.
- *Childhood gender nonconformity* refers to variation from norms in gender role behavior such as toy preferences, rough-and-tumble play, aggression, or playmate gender. The terms **gender variance** and **gender atypicality** have been used equivalently in the literature.
- *Gender discordance* refers to a discrepancy between anatomical sex and gender identity. The term **gender identity variance** has been used to denote a spectrum of gender discordant phenomena in the literature.

- ○ *Transgender* people have a gender identity that is discordant from their anatomical sex.
- ○ *Transsexuals* are transgender people who make their perceived gender and/or anatomical sex conform with their gender identity through strategies, such as dress, grooming, hormone use, and/or surgery (known as ***sex reassignment***).
- *Gender minority* refers to gender nonconforming and gender discordant children, adolescents, and adults.[3]

Stewart L. Adelson, MD
Department of Psychiatry
Columbia University College of Physicians and Surgeons
Department of Psychiatry
Weill Cornell Medical College
New York, NY 10032, USA

Nadia L. Dowshen, MD
Gender and Sexuality Development Clinic
Craig-Dalsimer Division of Adolescent Medicine
PolicyLab
Children's Hospital of Philadelphia
Perelman School of Medicine
University of Pennsylvania
34th Street & Civic Center Boulevard
Philadelphia, PA 19104, USA

Harvey J. Makadon, MD, FACP
The Fenway Institute
Harvard Medical School
Ansin Building
1340 Boylston Street
Boston, MA 02215, USA

Robert Garofalo, MD, MPH
Adolescent Medicine
Center for Gender, Sexuality, and HIV Prevention
Ann & Robert H. Lurie Children's Hospital of Chicago
Northwestern University Feinberg School of Medicine
303 East Chicago Avenue
Chicago, IL 60611, USA

E-mail addresses:
sla15@cumc.columbia.edu (S.L. Adelson)
dowshenn@email.chop.edu (N.L. Dowshen)
HMakadon@fenwayhealth.org (H.J. Makadon)
RGarofalo@luriechildrens.org (R. Garofalo)

REFERENCES

1. American Academy of Pediatrics Committee on Adolescence. Office-based care for lesbian, gay, bisexual, transgender, and questioning youth. Pediatrics 2013; 132(1):198–203.
2. Institute of Medicine (US), Committee on Lesbian, Gay, Bisexual, and Transgender Health Issues and Research Gaps and Opportunities. The health of lesbian, gay,

bisexual, and transgender people: building a foundation for better understanding. Washington (DC): National Academies Press (US); 2011.

3. Adelson SL, the American Academy of Child and Adolescent Psychiatry (AACAP) Committee on Quality Issues (CQI). Practice parameter on gay, lesbian or bisexual sexual orientation, gender-nonconformity, and gender discordance in children and adolescents. J Am Acad Child Adolesc Psychiatry 2012;51(9):957–74.

4. Coleman E, Bockting W, Botzer M, et al. Standards of care for the health of trans-sexual, transgender, and gender-nonconforming people, version 7. International Journal of Transgenderism 2011;13:165–232.

5. Meyer IH. Prejudice, social stress, and mental health in lesbian, gay, and bisexual populations: conceptual issues and research evidence. Psych Bull 2003;129(5): 674–97.

6. Herdt G, van de Meer T. Homophobia and Anti-Gay Violence–Contemporary Perspectives. Editorial introduction. Culture, Health & Sexuality 2003;5(2):99–101.

Erratum

An error was made in Pediatric Clinics of North America, Volume 62, Issue 2, April 2015, Pages 471–489. In the article, "Cardiac Evaluation of the Newborn," on page 841, the sentence "Because PaCO2 is a measure of oxygen dissolved in plasma, it is normal," should read 'PaO2' not PaCO2.

http://dx.doi.org/10.1016/j.pcl.2016.08.001
0031-3955/16/Published by Elsevier Inc.
pediatric.theclinics.com

Caring for Lesbian, Gay, Bisexual, Transgender, and Questioning Youth in Inclusive and Affirmative Environments

(●) CrossMark

Scott E. Hadland, MD, MPH, MS[a,b,]*, Baligh R. Yehia, MD, MPP, MSc[c,d],
Harvey J. Makadon, MD[e,f]

KEYWORDS

- Adolescents • Sexuality • Ambulatory care • Primary health care
- Reproductive health services

KEY POINTS

- Lesbian, gay, bisexual, transgender, queer and questioning (LGBTQ) youth may experience interpersonal and structural stigma within the health care environment.
- Inclusive and affirmative care for LGBTQ youth requires a careful understanding not only of the unique aspects of LGBTQ health care, but also of skills unique to caring for youth more generally.
- Although most LGBTQ youth are physically and mentally healthy, certain LGBTQ youth are at elevated risk of human immunodeficiency virus infection, sexually transmitted infection, pregnancy, obesity, substance use disorders, mood and anxiety disorders, eating disorders and other body image-related concerns, peer bullying, and family rejection.

Continued

Dr S.E. Hadland is supported by the Division of Adolescent and Young Adult Medicine at Boston Children's Hospital and the Leadership Education in Adolescent Health Training Program T71 MC00009 (Maternal and Child Health Bureau/Health Resources and Services Administration) and by a National Research Service Award 1T32 HD075727 (National Institutes of Health/National Institute of Child Health and Human Development).
Conflict of Interest Statement: The authors have nothing to disclose.

[a] Division of Adolescent/Young Adult Medicine, Department of Medicine, Boston Children's Hospital, 300 Longwood Avenue, Boston, MA 02115, USA; [b] Department of Pediatrics, Harvard Medical School, 25 Shattuck Street, Boston, MA 02115, USA; [c] Department of Medicine, Perelman School of Medicine, University of Pennsylvania, 1021 Blockley Hall, 423 Guardian Drive, Philadelphia, PA 19104, USA; [d] Penn Medicine Program for LGBT Health, Perelman School of Medicine, University of Pennsylvania, 1021 Blockley Hall, 423 Guardian Drive, Philadelphia, PA 19104, USA; [e] The Fenway Institute, Fenway Health, 1340 Boylston Street, Boston, MA 02215, USA; [f] Department of Medicine, Harvard Medical School, 25 Shattuck Street, Boston, MA 02115, USA
* Corresponding author. Division of Adolescent/Young Adult Medicine, Boston Children's Hospital, 300 Longwood Avenue, Boston, MA 02115.
E-mail address: scott.hadland@childrens.harvard.edu

Pediatr Clin N Am 63 (2016) 955–969
http://dx.doi.org/10.1016/j.pcl.2016.07.001

Continued

- Health care systems should be mindful of the availability, accessibility, acceptability, and equity of their services with regard to LGBTQ youth.
- Large-scale system changes to improve care for LGBTQ youth can be daunting to a health care organization, but some solutions can be adopted rapidly by individual providers and clinic staff and may be as simple as changing one's language and approach.

Lesbian, gay, bisexual, transgender, queer, and questioning (LGBTQ) youth, a group including nonheterosexual, gender-nonconforming, and gender-dysphoric children, adolescents, and young adults on multiple developmental trajectories toward LGBT adulthood, are more likely than their peers to experience stigma in the health care environment.[1,2] Providing care that is affirming and inclusive, that is, care that draws on knowledge and skills enabling a health care provider to work effectively with LGBTQ youth, is critical to improve health outcomes and quality.[2–4] The broader clinical environment, clinic flow and other organization functions, and administrative systems also need to be considered so as to ensure that clinical services are welcoming. Increasingly, examining these components and the messages they send to LGBTQ youth is not simply good care, but should be the baseline standard that health care organizations apply.[5] This is particularly important because prevalence estimates reveal that LGBTQ youth are inevitably a part of every general medical practice, whether providers realize it or not.[6]

This article begins by reviewing special considerations for the care of LGBTQ youth, then turns to systems-level principles underlying inclusive and affirming care. It then examines specific strategies that individual providers can use to provide more patient-centered care, and concludes with a discussion of how clinics and health systems can tailor clinical services to the needs of LGBTQ youth.

SPECIAL CONSIDERATIONS IN LESBIAN, GAY, BISEXUAL, TRANSGENDER, AND QUESTIONING YOUTH CARE

Ensuring high-quality care for LGBTQ youth requires providers to understand principles of caring for LGBTQ individuals as well as those of caring for young people more generally. Although most LGBTQ youth are physically and mentally healthy, certain LGBTQ youth are at elevated risk of human immunodeficiency virus (HIV) infection, sexually transmitted infection (STI), pregnancy, obesity, substance use disorders, mood and anxiety disorders, eating disorders and other body image-related concerns, peer bullying (see Valerie A. Earnshaw and colleagues' article, "LGBT Youth and Bullying," in this issue) and family rejection (see Sabra L. Katz-Wise and colleagues' article, "LGBT Youth and Family Acceptance," in this issue).[1,7] LGBTQ youth may avoid seeking health care due to fear of discrimination, and even once in care, may fear disclosure of their sexual orientation or gender identity and therefore withhold truthful responses from their health care providers.[1] Transgender youth face the added burden of locating providers with sufficient knowledge, competence, and experience to affirm their gender identity.[8,9] LGBTQ youth are also disproportionately more likely to be homeless,[10] and in many cases, this may be due to parental rejection or other trauma.[11]

Critical to understanding care of LGBTQ individuals and underlying many of these health disparities is stigma (see Mark L. Hatzenbeuhler's and John E. Pachankis' article, "Stigma and Minority Stress as Social Determinants of Health Among LGBT Youth: Research Evidence and Clinical Implications," in this issue).[12,13] Stigma is defined as the labeling of a specific group, and associated stereotyping, separation, status loss, and discrimination.[13,14] Both interpersonal (ie, stigma between patients and other people, which in the health care setting may include providers and other clinic staff) and structural stigma (ie, stigma resulting from systems and organizations, which in the health care setting may include the clinical environment, clinic flow, and other functions) have been barriers to inclusive and affirmative care for this population.[12,13,15,16]

As an example of how stigma affects the health of youth, rejection of an LGBTQ individual by his or her parents (see Sabra L. Katz-Wise and colleagues' article, "LGBT Youth and Family Acceptance," in this issue) may lead to separation and isolation, loss of resources (such as housing, food, clothing, and money), disadvantaged financial and social status, and ongoing discrimination. The links to social determinants of health (such as homelessness and poverty) and to adverse health outcomes (such as mood and anxiety problems, and substance use and related harms) are obvious. Stigma adversely affects LGBTQ youth, and is perpetuated in some health care settings. This is perhaps not surprising given the current lack of attention to educating medical students, trainees, and clinicians about issues related to LGBTQ health.[17,18]

Ensuring inclusive and affirmative health care environments for LGBTQ youth also requires in-depth understanding of general issues pertinent to caring for *all* children, adolescents, and young adults.[19] Youth have unique physiologic, neurocognitive, and psychosocial needs; accordingly, their care should be developmentally appropriate to these. Appropriate handling of youths' confidentiality is important; when sensitive information is disclosed by LGBTQ youth, it is a matter of paramount importance, discussed later in this article.[20] For youth in the process of transition from pediatric to adult clinical services, care can become fragmented.[21,22]

Youth often use language pertaining to sexual orientation and gender identity that may be unfamiliar to health care providers. Currently, there is expansive thinking about both sexual orientation and gender identity, particularly among youth. Many in the LGBTQ community even reject the terms lesbian, gay, bisexual, and transgender as not capturing all sexual orientations or gender identities.[23] For example, many youth describe themselves as queer, an umbrella term inclusive of all nonheterosexual sexual orientations and non–cis-gender identities. Some youth describe themselves as pansexual, asexual, or aromantic regarding sexual orientation. Gender identity is often thought of as outside the traditional male-female binary and on a spectrum; many youth self-describe as gender-nonconforming (defined in this issue as nonconformity in gender role expression, but sometimes used by youth differently to refer to gender identity variance) and use terms such as "gender-queer" or "gender-nonbinary." These issues, and how providers and their organizations can address them to generate LGBTQ youth-affirming clinical services, are outlined in subsequent sections.

SYSTEMS-LEVEL PRINCIPLES UNDERLYING LESBIAN, GAY, BISEXUAL, TRANSGENDER, AND QUESTIONING YOUTH-FRIENDLY SERVICES

The World Health Organization and other leading professional organizations have highlighted principles that should underlie all youth-friendly care,[19,24–26] and in addition, there are a number of technical reports and clinical practice guidelines to help clinicians apply these principles specifically to the care of LGBTQ youth.[1,5,27,28] Recognizing the unique biological, developmental, and psychosocial needs of children, adolescents, and young adults, and especially those who are LGBTQ, health services for youth should be optimized with regard to *availability*, *accessibility*, *acceptability*, and *equity*.[19]

Availability refers to the presence of health care providers with knowledge, competence, and experience working with young people with current or developing LGBTQ identities, feelings, or behavior. Accessibility is the relative ease with which LGBTQ youth can obtain care from an available provider. Acceptability is the extent to which clinical services are culturally competent and developmentally appropriate for LGBTQ youth, and as a critical component of this, the degree to which parents are involved when appropriate (especially in the care of younger children) and confidentiality is ensured and protected with youth while maintaining collaborative relationships that include appropriate boundaries with parents, other guardians, community members like school personnel, and colleagues. Equity refers to the extent to which clinical care and services are friendly to all LGBTQ youth, regardless of sexual orientation, gender expression, gender identity, race, ethnicity, language, ability to pay, housing status, and insurance status, among other factors. Each of these principles is reviewed in the following sections and summarized in **Table 1**.

Availability

Availability of LGBTQ youth-friendly services in many locales is limited by access to a workforce of health care providers with experience working with youth and LGBTQ populations.[27,29,30] This workforce includes a wide range of disciplines, including physicians, nurses, psychologists, social workers, dieticians, clinical assistants, community workers, clerical staff, and other professionals involved in health care delivery. The existing LGBTQ youth-friendly workforce is currently concentrated in urban areas and may be nonexistent in some rural and other locales.[31,32]

Even where clinical services for LGBTQ youth are available, quality of care may vary if patients and their caretakers do not receive the full set of recommended physical and mental health screening services, anticipatory guidance, and treatment.[27,28,33–37] For example, *Chlamydia trachomatis* screening for the general adolescent population has shown wide provider variability in adherence to recommended screening practices.[38,39] Although well-established clinical practice guidelines exist for providers caring for LGBTQ youth,[27,28,37] such guidelines are relatively new and there is likely to be wide variability in receipt of recommended screening and interventions across health care settings. Furthermore, as new knowledge emerges (as is often the case in the rapidly evolving field of LGBTQ youth health care), providers are likely to require ongoing training to remain up to date. Therefore, ensuring the availability of the full range of appropriate clinical services should not be viewed as a static, binary outcome that is either present or absent, but rather as a continuous process subject to ongoing measurement and quality improvement.[40]

Accessibility

Even where appropriate health services exist and where practices adhere to guidelines, providers should consider the accessibility of their services, not only with regard to the physical location, but also with regard to ease of entry into such services. LGBTQ adolescent and young adult-friendly services should be located near where LGBTQ youth live, study, or work, and should be accessible by public transportation or with free or low-cost parking.[19] In particular, LGBTQ youth may congregate in certain parts of cities or towns that are more LGBT-friendly, and locating clinical services nearby may be a logical choice.[2,41] Because LGBTQ youth are disproportionately likely to be homeless,[10] considering where and how homeless youth access health services is also critical and should take into consideration locations that homeless youth are likely to be present. In some cities, services are provided by a mobile van that travels to particular locations to maximize accessibility.[42]

Table 1
Systems-level principles underlying lesbian, gay, bisexual, transgender, questioning (LGBTQ) youth-friendly services

Principle	Definition	Examples
Availability	The presence of health care providers with knowledge, competence, and experience working with young people and with people with current or possibly developing LGBTQ identities, feelings, and/or behavior	• Providers from various disciplines (eg, physicians and nonphysician health care professionals) provide care sensitive to the needs of LGBTQ youth • Quality of care is high, with LGBTQ youth (and when appropriate, their caregivers) universally receiving recommended screening and anticipatory guidance
Accessibility	The relative ease with which LGBTQ youth can obtain care from an available provider	• Clinical services are located near where LGBTQ youth live, study, work, or otherwise spend time • Clinical services are easily obtained, with expanded hours during evenings and weekends, same-day urgent bookings, drop-in visits, allowances for late appointments • Technology (eg, online patient portals, e-mail, telemedicine) is increasingly used to improve access for youth
Acceptability	The extent to which clinical services are culturally competent and developmentally appropriate for LGBTQ youth, and to which confidentiality is ensured and protected	• The clinic has a policy affirming its inclusive services for LGBTQ, and the clinical environment has signs, stickers, and other statements showing it is LGBT-friendly • Health brochures and other reading materials are tailored to the needs of LGBTQ youth • Confidentiality is ensured and protected in every patient encounter and health care providers spend time one-on-one with patients to elicit sensitive information
Equity	The degree to which clinical care is friendly to *all* LGBTQ youth, regardless of race, ethnicity, language, ability to pay, housing status, and insurance status, among other factors	• High-quality care is provided to all youth, regardless of whether they are lesbian, gay, bisexual, or transgender • Culturally competent care is provided to LGBTQ youth of color and services are available for patients who are not native English speaking • Services are provided free-of-charge for uninsured LGBTQ youth

Adapted from Tylee A, Haller DM, Graham T, et al. Youth-friendly primary-care services: how are we doing and what more needs to be done? Lancet 2007;369(9572):1565–73; and Department of Maternal Newborn Child and Adolescent Health. Making health services adolescent friendly—developing national quality standards for adolescent friendly health services. Geneva (Switzerland): World Health Organization; 2012.

Where conveniently located, health care providers should ensure optimal accessibility in how adolescents obtain services. A critical component of the patient-centered medical home[43] is "enhanced access,"[44,45] which entails offering expanded hours during evenings and weekends,[46] same-day urgent care appointments,[47,48] drop-in visits,[49] and allowances for patients who arrive late for appointments.[50,51] Increasingly, youth and their caretakers are likely to expect Internet-based scheduling and communication with health care providers through e-mail or even telemedicine, where allowable.[52–55]

Acceptability

Especially salient in the care of LGBTQ youth is ensuring that even when services are available and accessible, clinical services have acceptability. Often, improving acceptability requires assessing the clinical environment and understanding ways that it can become more welcoming for and supportive of LGBTQ youth and families. For example, health brochures and other written materials available in the clinic should not assume heterosexuality, and certain topics, particularly safe sex, reproductive health, intimate partner relationship safety, family acceptance, and bullying, should be tailored to address the unique needs of LGBTQ youth.[2]

Traditional bathrooms can be very problematic for transgender youth.[56] For clinics with single-occupancy bathrooms, clinics should avoid labeling them as "male" or "female," or have an explicit, readily visible policy allowing youth to choose the bathroom that matches their identified gender rather than their biologic sex. For clinics with shared bathrooms, clinics should allow youth to choose the bathroom that matches their identified gender with a highly visible policy statement, and consider installing stalls with walls that reach to the floor for greater privacy.

More than simply identifying and eliminating potential barriers to care for LGBTQ youth, clinical leadership should be proactive about creating an affirming and inclusive environment for LGBTQ youth. This starts with the most fundamental aspect of a clinic: its mission statement.[2,5] Whether a clinic serves a large population of LGBTQ youth or the broader general adolescent population, it should explicitly state that it is welcoming, inclusive, and affirming of all youth with regard to sexual orientation, gender expression, and gender identity. To reinforce the mission statement and make clear that the clinical environment is welcoming to LGBTQ youth, signs and stickers might be placed in several well-trafficked locations (eg, rainbows or other widely understood symbols in clinic check-in areas and examination rooms). Providers might wear lapel pins or lanyards that reaffirm these messages to show that they as an individual clinician also seek to provide care sensitive to the needs of LGBTQ youth. These approaches establish an environment that reduces interpersonal and structural stigma and promotes a safe clinical space for LGBTQ youth.

Providing appropriately confidential clinical services for LGBTQ youth is central to achieving acceptability, because fear of a breach of privacy is a common reason that adolescents avoid seeking care.[20,57] Approaches individual providers should take to protect confidentiality are discussed later in this article.

Equity

Finally, medical care has not been universally equitable for LGBTQ youth.[58,59] To achieve true equity, it must be provided to all groups of lesbian, gay, bisexual, transgender, queer, and questioning youth. For example, providers may have competence in working with gay, lesbian, or bisexual youth, but may not feel comfortable or have comparable experience in caring for transgender and gender-nonconforming youth.[60,61] Providers also need to ensure that services are inclusive of and sensitive to the needs of diverse racial/ethnic groups of LGBTQ youth, including those of color and those who are not native English speaking.[62] Finally, providers should ensure that services are provided to all LGBTQ youth regardless of ability to pay. Many youth, particularly those without legal immigrant status in the United States, without health insurance, or without stable housing are likely to have unmet health needs.[63–65] LGBTQ youth who have been rejected by their families are especially at risk of being uninsured and homeless. Through public entitlements, grants, or other funding opportunities, providers should attempt to provide free or low-cost services to LGBTQ youth who are unable to pay for clinical services.

STRATEGIES FOR INDIVIDUAL PROVIDERS

Large-scale system changes can be daunting to a health care organization seeking to improve its care for LGBTQ youth. However, some solutions can be adopted more rapidly by providers and clinic staff and may be as simple as changing one's language and approach. Specific strategies to make a clinic more inclusive and affirming for LGBTQ youth that are more immediately available to providers and their organizations are summarized in **Box 1**.

Confidentiality

Establishing and safeguarding confidentiality with youth as a crucial element of a safe, viable treatment relationship, concomitantly with maintaining collaborative relationships that include developmentally appropriate privacy from adult parents or guardians, school personnel, colleagues, and other important adults in the youth's life, is critical in the care of *all* youth, but especially so for LGBTQ youth. At the beginning of every encounter, providers should verify that confidentiality has been appropriately explained, ensured, and fully protected in a manner consistent with applicable pediatric guidelines and ethics. Doing so is standard of care,[38,39] and is especially important for youth who have not yet disclosed any nonheterosexual attractions, behavior, or identity or gender-variant identity to family or friends.[38,39] Improper disclosure of such details could damage the patient-provider relationship and lead to physical or emotional harm if caretakers or others have a negative reaction. Thus, information on sexual orientation and gender identity should be especially carefully protected.[20,24,33,36] Although in certain clinical situations (such as suicidal ideation, homicidal ideation, or suspicion of abuse or neglect) local law may require disclosure to the parent or guardian of a minor patient, it may at the same time allow or require providers to protect a youth's confidentiality of sexual and reproductive health concerns throughout treatment.[20] Therefore, any mandatory disclosures should be handled in a way that discloses only the minimum information necessary to ensure immediate safety and preserves remaining confidentiality. In addition to protecting youth and preserving the clinical relationship with them, it may also improve the accuracy of youths' responses to questions about risk behaviors and other sensitive topics, because they may feel more comfortable disclosing personal information.[66] Clinicians also should maintain confidentiality in medical records (both handwritten and electronic) by specific indications in clinical notes regarding any portions that are not to be shared with parents or guardians.[20]

For youth who are accompanied by a parent or guardian at their visit, the provider should ensure he or she spends time alone one-on-one with the patient.[20,36] The provider can then update the parent on nonconfidential aspects of care that the patient agrees to share. In some cases, providers may be instrumental in engaging families in difficult conversations regarding sexual orientation or gender identity if the patient wishes.

Box 1
Specific strategies for providers to create a welcoming environment for lesbian, gay, bisexual, transgender, and questioning (LGBTQ) youth

Language	Use words that help establish a trusting relationship; avoid words that build barriers to care. Language and word choice is critical not only in your clinical encounter, but also in all communication with nurses, clinical assistants, front desk staff, and all other staff.

- Avoid assuming a patient's partner is opposite-sex. Ask, "Are you in a relationship?" rather than, "Do you have a boyfriend?"
- Use the same terms youth use to describe themselves. If a patient refers to himself as "gay," use this instead of the term "homosexual" in your clinical encounter.
- Ask what pronouns a patient prefers, then use them. Transgender males, for example, may prefer that you use the terms, "he," "him," and "his." Other youth may use gender-neutral terms such as "they" or "zie."

Expectations	Be aware that LGBTQ youth may have had prior adverse health care interactions and may not immediately feel comfortable disclosing sensitive information to you.

- Up front, let your patient know that you are an LGBT-friendly provider. Many clinics will post materials on the walls stating that they are LGBT-friendly; often, providers will wear a rainbow pin or other affirming symbol to let youth know they welcome LGBTQ youth at their practice.
- At the beginning of every social history, state, "With your permission, I'd like to ask you some questions that I ask of all the youth I care for."
- Always discuss confidentiality and ensure it with all youth. If a patient comes with a parent, always ensure one-on-one confidential time with youth. Explain confidentiality to parents, also, so they understand that you will not disclose certain aspects of care.

Questions	Understand that LGBTQ youth may have diverse and fluid identities with regard to sexual attraction, self-identified sexual orientation, gender identity, and gender expression.

- Ask open-ended questions about preferred pronouns, gender identity, self-identified sexual orientation, and sexual attraction, and only when one-on-one with youth.
- Understand that the labels youth use do not necessarily dictate a youth's sexual partners and associated sexual behaviors. Understanding who a patient's partners are even despite the labels youth use can help guide clinical care.

Barriers	Understand that navigating health care systems can be frustrating, and LGBTQ youth experience the same barriers to care as other youth, and more.

- Some barriers to care, such as insurance problems, are common among all youth, but may be especially common for LGBTQ youth who in some cases may be estranged from their families; be prepared to offer assistance with insurance problems and where necessary, free-of-charge services

Charting	Be aware that health care records and insurance plans often use the name a patient was assigned at birth, which can be problematic for transgender youth who have changed their name. The gender listed often reflects a patient's assigned gender at birth.

- Consider a special chart-labeling system or identify a feature in your electronic medical record that identifies patients by their chosen name.
- Determine whether your medical record system can include fields not only for "male" or "female," but also for "transgender male" or "transgender female," as appropriate.
- Review the forms your clinic mails to patients or administers in the waiting room. Often, these contain binary male/female fields, but should include other options as well.

Handling mistakes	Know that even experienced practitioners sometimes make mistakes with names and pronouns. Be prepared to correct them when they occur.
	• Confront head-on your own mistakes or those of your colleagues when they occur. To a transgender female called her assigned male birth name by a clinic staff member, say, "I apologize that we used the wrong name for you. We strive to be respectful of all our patients and we did not mean to disrespect you."
	• Hold all staff accountable for creating a welcoming environment, starting at the front desk and proceeding to every clinic staff worker. Work to improve the quality of your organization's care by making an LGBTQ youth-friendly environment a priority and discuss it openly and frequently with staff.

Adapted from National LGBTQ Health Education Center. Providing welcoming services and care for LGBTQ people. Boston: The Fenway Institute; 2015; with permission.

Despite efforts to ensure confidentiality, some patients may not feel comfortable honestly answering direct questions regarding sexuality, gender nonconformity and/or gender identity, or related peer or family difficulties from the clinician, and using collateral or alternative information sources (including electronic or other forms of screening before the visit or in the waiting room) may help LGBTQ youth provide more honest responses to these and other sensitive topics.[67,68] Unfortunately, for youth who are on parents' insurance plans, explanations of benefit (EOBs) can sometimes reveal confidential care (eg, STI screening and/or treatment). There are currently efforts in some states to limit insurance companies' communication of such confidential information to primary policyholders.[69] Thus, it is important for clinicians to consider that inadvertent disclosure of sensitive clinical details can occur when they order laboratory tests or prescribe medications for STIs, and should plan accordingly. In some cases, offering care free-of-charge may be the only way to avoid accidental disclosure through EOBs; in some locales, use of special grant funds allows providers to offer free and confidential testing and treatment that avoid the need to bill patients' insurance. Clinicians should bear similar issues in mind when making a plan for delivering test results after an encounter or when writing or approving prescriptions, as well as when they are dispensed.

STRATEGIES FOR CLINICS AND HEALTH SYSTEMS

The principles and strategies outlined previously are important general approaches to improving the friendliness of clinical care for LGBTQ youth; however, delivering affirmative care may require moving past a one-size-fits-all approach and exploring the specific needs of the LGBTQ youth population of a clinic or health system. For example, the needs of a clinic serving primarily gay and lesbian youth is likely to be very different from one serving primarily transgender youth. Clinics serving young LGBTQ adults are likely to face different clinical scenarios from those who treat primarily younger adolescents. The needs of rural LGBTQ youth may be quite different from those of urban LGBTQ youth. Children who are or may be growing up as LGBTQ can and do live everywhere. Although core clinical practice guidelines exist and should be adhered to, clinics should explore the needs of their own population so as to develop and improve the services they offer LGBTQ youth. Here, we discuss approaches to assessing the needs of the population that a clinic serves.

Readiness Assessment

As highlighted previously, providers can make a number of small, easily accomplished changes to substantially improve the inclusiveness of their clinical services for LGBTQ youth. However, some clinics or health systems may seek to create broader changes and should first consider a readiness assessment that combines an analysis of population health data with qualitative study methods.[2,14] For example, in evaluating their own population health data, a clinic might examine its rates of positive STI screens to understand which youth are most likely to test positive, and consider how best to deliver health services to those youth. However, examination of population health data alone is likely to lead to excessive focus on adverse health outcomes to the exclusion of positive health behaviors that clinicians might promote.[70] Additionally, population health data alone are unlikely to fully describe patient satisfaction and experience of care, including highlighting ways in which LGBTQ youth may experience stigma in the health care environment.[2,13]

Therefore, clinics should supplement their study of population health data with qualitative methods in their needs assessment.[70] Methodologic approaches might include focus groups of LGBTQ youth, or if younger adolescents are to be interviewed or there are confidentiality concerns, one-on-one interviews.[71] Parents should also be engaged, either in their own separate focus groups or in interviews. Key informant interviews with community stakeholders (eg, community workers and other service providers, educators, and faith leaders) should also be conducted to understand how LGBTQ youth interface with the world beyond the clinic's walls.

Questions for youth, families, and stakeholders should focus on all aspects of the care experience and examine the systems-level principles outlined earlier (availability, accessibility, acceptability, and equity),[19,24] as well as individual provider-level characteristics. Details considered might include clinic location, hours, services (including low-cost or free and confidential preventive screening, treatment and referral), costs, mission statement, facilities, signage (including evidence of LGBTQ friendliness), educational materials, confidentiality, and perceived inclusiveness for youth of color.[19,25] Providers should also consider the extent to which they might bolster outside services to aid youth in the broader community (eg, help with housing and other social services, legal support, help with employment searches, and collaborations with schools, faith-based organizations, and other community organizations). The advantage to this approach is that clinics leveraging community programs do not need to necessarily duplicate such services within their own walls.

Such a needs assessment is likely to uncover unanticipated ways that a clinic might better serve its LGBTQ youth population. Not only should the needs assessment serve to help providers understand new services they might develop or preexisting services they might improve, but it also should help clinical leadership understand new measures for quality improvement.[72] For example, one process measure might be asking all patients about sexual orientation and gender identity or about a preferred name and pronouns for the youth, and recording this in a prominent place in the patient care flow (for youth comfortable with this information being freely available) or in a confidential part of the electronic medical record (for youth who wish to maintain the privacy of this information). Youth might also help providers develop LGBTQ youth-specific patient satisfaction measures for the clinic.[26] Each clinic should let the needs and requests of their own clinic population drive the development of quality measures, and ensure that such measures are frequently assessed to drive ongoing improvement.

Training

Many clinics choose to offer training on competent care for LGBTQ youth to their clinic staff. Trainings can be offered as an in-person workshop, or where such workshops are not readily available, online webinars offer excellent convenience (eg, http://www.lgbthealtheducation.org/training/on-demand-webinars/). Training is available in both cultural and clinical competence. Some aspects of cultural competence training are appropriate for *all* clinic staff (including front desk and other administrative staff), such as proper use of pronouns and preferred names, to ensure competence at every moment of the care experience.[56] Clinical competence trainings, such as those reviewing clinical practice guidelines for the care of LGBTQ youth,[27,28,37,73] are more appropriate for clinicians. Such trainings may be critical given the lack of formal medical education on LGBTQ health care otherwise available to many providers, particularly those who trained some time ago.[17] Providers and clinics might consider reaching out to local organizations who serve youth in the community or to other nearby health care providers with expertise in serving LGBTQ youth to help arrange trainings.

SUMMARY

Reevaluating and redesigning systems of care and individual provider practices to improve clinical services for LGBTQ youth should be a priority for health care organizations.[5] Some changes, such as changing the language clinic staff use when working with LGBTQ youth, can be put into practice immediately with minimal overhaul of clinical services. Others require a more in-depth readiness assessment and reorganization of preexisting practices. However, the up-front investment is likely to pay off for both patients and providers. Based on population estimates, *all* general medical providers are likely already caring for LGBTQ youth but may not realize it because youth are struggling with their own identity or may not be ready to disclose.[6] It is not the task of the provider to identify LGBTQ youth, but rather to ask appropriate questions and signal support for when youth are ready to disclose, and then offer further support and resources. LGBTQ youth are especially susceptible to stigma and discrimination in the traditional health care setting and yet have important physical and mental health care needs. Realizing the goal of creating a welcoming, inclusive, and affirming health care environment can improve health care outcomes for this historically marginalized group and create a rewarding practice for providers.

REFERENCES

1. Institute of Medicine. The health of lesbian, gay, bisexual, and transgender people: building a foundation for better understanding. Washington, DC: The National Academies Press; 2011.
2. Wilkerson JM, Rybicki S, Barber CA, et al. Creating a culturally competent clinical environment for LGBT patients. J Gay Lesb Soc Serv 2011;23(3):376–94.
3. Schultz D. Cultural competence in psychosocial and psychiatric care: a critical perspective with reference to research and clinical experiences in California, US and in Germany. Soc Work Health Care 2004;39(3–4):231–47.
4. Yehia BR, Calder D, Flesch JD, et al. Advancing LGBT health at an academic medical center: a case study. LGBT Health 2014;2(4):362–6.
5. Human Rights Campaign Foundation Health & Aging Program. Healthcare Equality Index 2014: promoting equitable and inclusive care for lesbian, gay,

bisexual and transgender patients and their families. Washington, DC: Human Rights Campaign Foundation; 2014.

6. Kann L, Kinchen S, Shanklin SL, et al. Youth risk behavior surveillance–United States, 2013. MMWR Surveill Summ 2014;63(Suppl 4):1–168.

7. Agwu AL, Lee L, Fleishman JA, et al. Aging and loss to follow-up among youth living with human immunodeficiency virus in the HIV Research Network. J Adolesc Health 2015;56(3):345–51.

8. Rachlin K, Green J, Lombardi E. Utilization of health care among female-to-male transgender individuals in the United States. J Homosex 2008;54(3):243–58.

9. Sanchez NF, Sanchez JP, Danoff A. Health care utilization, barriers to care, and hormone usage among male-to-female transgender persons in New York City. Am J Public Health 2009;99(4):713–9.

10. Corliss HL, Goodenow CS, Nichols L, et al. High burden of homelessness among sexual-minority adolescents: findings from a representative Massachusetts high school sample. Am J Public Health 2011;101(9):1683–9.

11. Whitbeck LB, Chen X, Hoyt DR, et al. Mental disorder, subsistence strategies, and victimization among gay, lesbian, and bisexual homeless and runaway adolescents. J Sex Res 2004;41(4):329–42.

12. Hatzenbuehler ML. How does sexual minority stigma "get under the skin"? A psychological mediation framework. Psychol Bull 2009;135(5):707.

13. Hatzenbuehler ML, Phelan JC, Link BG. Stigma as a fundamental cause of population health inequalities. Am J Public Health 2013;103(5):813–21.

14. Link BG, Phelan JC. Conceptualizing stigma. Annu Rev Sociol 2001;27:363–85.

15. Hatzenbuehler ML, Bellatorre A, Lee Y, et al. Structural stigma and all-cause mortality in sexual minority populations. Soc Sci Med 2014;103:33–41.

16. Metzl JM, Hansen H. Structural competency: theorizing a new medical engagement with stigma and inequality. Soc Sci Med 2014;103:126–33.

17. Obedin-Maliver J, Goldsmith ES, Stewart L, et al. Lesbian, gay, bisexual, and transgender–related content in undergraduate medical education. JAMA 2011; 306(9):971–7.

18. Makadon HJ. Improving health care for the lesbian and gay communities. N Engl J Med 2006;354(9):895–7.

19. Tylee A, Haller DM, Graham T, et al. Youth-friendly primary-care services: how are we doing and what more needs to be done? Lancet 2007;369(9572):1565–73.

20. Ford C, English A, Sigman G. Confidential health care for adolescents: position paper for the Society for Adolescent Medicine. J Adolesc Health 2004;35(2):160–7.

21. Cooley WC, Sagerman PJ. Supporting the health care transition from adolescence to adulthood in the medical home. Pediatrics 2011;128(1):182–200.

22. Yehia BR, Kangovi S, Frank I. Patients in transition: avoiding detours on the road to HIV treatment success. AIDS 2013;27(10):1529–33.

23. Kuper LE, Nussbaum R, Mustanski B. Exploring the diversity of gender and sexual orientation identities in an online sample of transgender individuals. J Sex Res 2012;49(2–3):244–54.

24. Department of Maternal Newborn Child and Adolescent Health. Making health services adolescent friendly—developing national quality standards for adolescent friendly health services. Geneva (Switzerland): World Health Organization; 2012.

25. Haller DM, Sanci LA, Patton GC, et al. Toward youth friendly services: a survey of young people in primary care. J Gen Intern Med 2007;22(6):775–81.

26. Ambresin A-E, Bennett K, Patton GC, et al. Assessment of youth-friendly health care: a systematic review of indicators drawn from young people's perspectives. J Adolesc Health 2013;52(6):670–81.

27. Society for Adolescent Health and Medicine. Recommendations for promoting the health and well-being of lesbian, gay, bisexual, and transgender adolescents: a position paper of the Society for Adolescent Health and Medicine. J Adolesc Health 2013;52(4):506–10.

28. Levine DA. Office-based care for lesbian, gay, bisexual, transgender, and questioning youth. Pediatrics 2013;132(1):e297–313.

29. Kim WJ. Child and adolescent psychiatry workforce: a critical shortage and national challenge. Acad Psychiatry 2003;27(4):277–82.

30. Hergenroeder AC, Benson PAS, Britto MT, et al. Adolescent medicine: workforce trends and recommendations. Arch Pediatr Adolesc Med 2010;164(12):1086–90.

31. Fisher CM, Irwin JA, Coleman JD. LGBT health in the Midlands: a rural/urban comparison of basic health indicators. J Homosex 2014;61(8):1062–90.

32. Lewis MK, Marshall I. Urban and rural challenges. In: LGBT psychology. Springer; 2012. p. 155–73.

33. Elster AB, Kuznets NJ. AMA Guidelines for Adolescent Preventive Services (GAPS): Recommendations and Rationale. Baltimore (MD): Williams & Wilkins; 1994.

34. American Academy of Family Physicians. Summary of recommendations for clinical preventive services. Leawood (KS); 2015.

35. Irwin CE, Adams SH, Park MJ, et al. Preventive care for adolescents: few get visits and fewer get services. Pediatrics 2009;123(4):e565–72.

36. American Academy of Pediatrics, Bright Futures Steering Committee. Adolescence (11 to 21 Years). In: Hagan JF, Shaw JS, Duncan PM, editors. Bright Futures: Guidelines for Health Supervision of Infants, Children, and Adolescents. 3rd edition. Elk Grove Village (IL): American Academy of Pediatrics; 2008. p. 155–68.

37. Adelson SL, American Academy of Child and Adolescent Psychiatry (AACAP) Committee on Quality Issues (CQI). Practice parameter on gay, lesbian or bisexual sexual orientation, gender-nonconformity, and gender discordance in children and adolescents. J Am Acad Child Adolesc Psychiatry 2012;51(9): 957–74.

38. Shafer M-AB, Tebb KP, Pantell RH, et al. Effect of a clinical practice improvement intervention on chlamydial screening among adolescent girls. JAMA 2002; 288(22):2846–52.

39. Tebb KP, Pantell RH, Wibbelsman CJ, et al. Screening sexually active adolescents for *Chlamydia trachomatis*: what about the boys? Am J Public Health 2005;95(10):1806–10.

40. Klein JD, Sesselberg TS, Gawronski B, et al. Improving adolescent preventive services through state, managed care, and community partnerships. J Adolesc Health 2003;32(6 Suppl):91–7.

41. Medeiros DM, Seehaus M, Elliott J, et al. Providing mental health services for LGBT teens in a community adolescent health clinic. J Gay Lesb Psychother 2004;8(3–4):83–95.

42. Woods ER, Samples CL, Melchiono MW, et al. Boston HAPPENS Program: A model of health care for HIV-positive, homeless, and at-risk youth. J Adolesc Heal 1998;23(2):37–48.

43. Yehia BR, Agwu AL, Schranz A, et al. Conformity of pediatric/adolescent HIV clinics to the patient-centered medical home care model. AIDS Patient Care STDS 2013;27(5):272–9.
44. National Committee for Quality Assurance. NCQA patient-centered medical home: improving experiences for patients, providers and practice staff. Washington, DC: National Committee for Quality Assurance; 2014.
45. Walker I, McManus MA, Fox HB. Medical home innovations: where do adolescents fit. Washington, DC: Natl Alliance Adv Adolesc Heal Rep 2011;(7).
46. Coker TR, Sareen HG, Chung PJ, et al. Improving access to and utilization of adolescent preventive health care: the perspectives of adolescents and parents. J Adolesc Health 2010;47(2):133–42.
47. Murray MM, Tantau C. Same-day appointments: exploding the access paradigm. Fam Pract Manag 2000;7(8):45.
48. Akinbami LJ, Gandhi H, Cheng TL. Availability of adolescent health services and confidentiality in primary care practices. Pediatrics 2003;111(2):394–401.
49. Newman BS, Passidomo K, Gormley K, et al. Use of drop-in clinic versus appointment-based care for LGBT youth: influences on the likelihood to access different health-care structures. LGBT Health 2014;1(2):140–6.
50. Institute for Healthcare Improvement. Shortening waiting times: six principles for improved access. 2014. Available at: http://www.ihi.org/resources/pages/improvementstories/shorteningwaitingtimessixprinciplesforimprovedaccess.aspx. Accessed September 28, 2015.
51. Ginsburg KR, Menapace AS, Slap GB. Factors affecting the decision to seek health care: the voice of adolescents. Pediatrics 1997;100(6):922–30.
52. Kleiner KD, Akers R, Burke BL, et al. Parent and physician attitudes regarding electronic communication in pediatric practices. Pediatrics 2002;109(5):740–4.
53. Anoshiravani A, Gaskin GL, Groshek MR, et al. Special requirements for electronic medical records in adolescent medicine. J Adolesc Health 2012;51(5):409–14.
54. Barlow E, Aggarwal A, Johnstone J, et al. Can paediatric and adolescent gynecological care be delivered via Telehealth? Paediatr Child Health 2012;17(2):e12.
55. Weaver B, Lindsay B, Gitelman B. Communication technology and social media: opportunities and implications for healthcare systems. Online J Issues Nurs 2012;17(3):3.
56. National LGBT Health Education Center/The Fenway Institute. Providing welcoming services and care for LGBT people: a learning guide for health care staff. Boston (MA): The Fenway Institute; 2015. Available at: http://www.lgbthealtheducation.org/wp-content/uploads/Learning-Guide.pdf. Accessed September 30, 2015.
57. Reddy DM, Fleming R, Swain C. Effect of mandatory parental notification on adolescent girls' use of sexual health care services. JAMA 2002;288(6):710–4.
58. Acevedo-Polakovich ID, Bell B, Gamache P, et al. Service accessibility for lesbian, gay, bisexual, transgender, and questioning youth. Youth Soc 2013;45(1):75–97.
59. Hoffman ND, Freeman K, Swann S. Healthcare preferences of lesbian, gay, bisexual, transgender and questioning youth. J Adolesc Health 2009;45(3):222–9.
60. Durso LE, Gates GJ. Serving Our Youth: Findings from a National Survey of Service Providers Working with Lesbian, Gay, Bisexual, and Transgender Youth who are Homeless or At Risk of Becoming Homeless. Los Angeles: The Williams Institute with True Colors Fund and The Palette Fund; 2012.

61. Knight RE, Shoveller JA, Carson AM, et al. Examining clinicians' experiences providing sexual health services for LGBTQ youth: considering social and structural determinants of health in clinical practice. Health Educ Res 2014;29(4): 662–70.
62. Kuper LE, Coleman BR, Mustanski BS. Coping with LGBT and racial–ethnic-related stressors: a mixed-methods study of LGBT youth of color. J Res Adolesc 2014;24(4):703–19.
63. Guendelman S, Angulo V, Wier M, et al. Overcoming the odds: access to care for immigrant children in working poor families in California. Matern Child Health J 2005;9(4):351–62.
64. Avila RM, Bramlett MD. Language and immigrant status effects on disparities in Hispanic children's health status and access to health care. Matern Child Health J 2013;17(3):415–23.
65. Yen S, Parmar DD, Lin EL, et al. Emergency contraception pill awareness and knowledge in uninsured adolescents: high rates of misconceptions concerning indications for use, side effects, and access. J Pediatr Adolesc Gynecol 2015; 28(5):337–42.
66. Ford CA, Millstein SG, Halpern-Felsher BL, et al. Influence of physician confidentiality assurances on adolescents' willingness to disclose information and seek future health care: a randomized controlled trial. JAMA 1997;278(12):1029–34.
67. Barbee LA, Dhanireddy S, Tat S, et al. 3 barriers to bacterial STI screening of HIV+ men who have sex with men (MSM) in HIV primary care settings. Sex Transm Infect 2013;89(Suppl 1):A41.
68. Cahill S, Makadon H. Sexual orientation and gender identity data collection in clinical settings and in electronic health records: a key to ending LGBT health disparities. LGBT Health 2014;1(1):34–41.
69. English A, Gold RB, Nash E, et al. Confidentiality for Individuals Insured as Dependents: A Review of State Laws and Policies. New York: Guttmacher Institute and Public Health Solutions; 2012. Available at http://www.guttmacher.org/pubs/confidentiality-review.pdf. Accessed September 30, 2015.
70. Wright J, Williams R, Wilkinson JR. Development and importance of health needs assessment. BMJ 1998;316(7140):1310–3.
71. Pope C, Ziebland S, Mays N. Qualitative research in health care. Analysing qualitative data. BMJ 2000;320(7227):114–6.
72. American Academy of Pediatrics. Enhancing pediatric workforce diversity and providing culturally effective pediatric care: implications for practice, education, and policy making. Pediatrics 2013;132(4):e1105–16.
73. Coleman E, Bockting W, Botzer M, et al. Standards of care for the health of transsexual, transgender, and gender-nonconforming people, version 7. Int J Transgend 2011;13:165–232.

Development and Mental Health of Lesbian, Gay, Bisexual, or Transgender Youth in Pediatric Practice

Stewart L. Adelson, MD[a,b,]*, Oliver M. Stroeh, MD[c], Yiu Kee Warren Ng, MD[d]

KEYWORDS

- Lesbian • Gay • Bisexual • Transgender • Child • Adolescent • Youth
- Mental health

KEY POINTS

- Mental health problems are leading causes of morbidity and mortality in all (not just lesbian, gay, bisexual, or transgender [LGBT]) youth.
- Pediatricians should monitor and support mental health in all youth.
- Like all youth, most LGBT youth are mentally healthy; however, their risk for mental health problems is somewhat elevated.
- Anti-LGBT stigma like social prejudice, peer bullying, family rejection, and self-nonacceptance are major risk factors.

INTRODUCTION

Mental health problems are highly prevalent in youth and are a significant cause of morbidity and mortality. For example, among adolescents and young adults in the United States, suicide is the third leading cause of mortality from age 10 to 14 years, and the second from age 15 to 24 years.[1] If left unaddressed, mental health problems

The authors have nothing to disclose.
[a] Department of Psychiatry, Division of Gender, Sexuality & Health and of Child & Adolescent Psychiatry, Columbia University College of Physicians & Surgeons, 117 West 17th Street, Ste. 2B, New York, NY 10011, USA; [b] Department of Psychiatry, Weill Cornell Medical College, New York, NY, USA; [c] Department of Psychiatry, Division of Child & Adolescent Psychiatry, Columbia University College of Physicians & Surgeons, New York State Psychiatric Institute, 1051 Riverside Drive, Unit #78, New York, NY 10032, USA; [d] Department of Psychiatry, Division of Child & Adolescent Psychiatry, Columbia University Medical Center, NYP-MSCH, 3959 Broadway CHONY North-6th Floor #629, New York, NY 10032, USA
* Corresponding author.
E-mail address: sla15@cumc.columbia.edu

like depression, anxiety, disruptive behavior, and learning problems can become chronic and cause serious morbidity; however, these can be significantly ameliorated by appropriate mental health interventions.[2] In addition to their inherent morbidity and mortality, psychiatric illnesses also may increase physical health risk behavior; for example, substance abuse (see Romulo Alcalde Aromin Jr's article, "Substance Abuse Prevention, Assessment and Treatment for LGBT Youth," in this issue) is associated with increased sexual risk behavior and exposure to sexually transmitted infections (STIs).[3] Therefore, these are very important problems for pediatricians to know about, recognize, and address.

Most youth with psychiatric diagnoses do not receive formal mental health treatment; as a result, mental health problems in children and adolescents are often encountered first by pediatricians.[2] The delay from the initial onset of symptoms until the start of mental health treatment can be years. According to the Agency for Healthcare Research and Quality (2009),[4] children's mental health disorders are among the top 5 most-costly medical conditions, costing the United States $8.9 billion annually. Therefore, pediatric primary care providers and other pediatric clinicians play a key role in detecting, assessing, and addressing youths' mental health needs.

Lesbian, gay, bisexual, or transgender (LGBT) youth have the same pediatric and developmental needs as the general population, as well as certain LGBT-specific health and mental health needs.[3,5,6] The ability to intervene appropriately when mental health problems exist, an important pediatric clinical competence in general, may be especially salient for youth who are or might be on a developmental path toward being LGBT. Although most lesbian, gay, and bisexual (LGB) youth are free from mental illness, a minority develops a psychiatric illness or has other mental health needs, like all youth.

The rates at which LGB youth experience certain mental illnesses, such as depression, anxiety, and substance abuse, are increased in comparison with the general population.[7] For example, they are at twofold to fivefold risk for suicidality.[8] This increase appears to be related to increased exposure to mental health stressors like peer harassment, bullying, and family rejection, specific problems that are addressed elsewhere in this issue (see Mark L. Hatzenbuehler and John E. Pachankis' article, "Stigma and Minority Stress as Social Determinants of Health Among LGBT Youth: Research Evidence and Clinical Implications"; Valerie A. Earnshaw and colleagues' article, "LGBT Youth and Bullying"; and Sabra L. Katz-Wise and colleagues' article, "LGBT Youth and Family Acceptance," in this issue). The mental health needs of youth diagnosed with gender dysphoria, who may be growing up to be transgender adults, remain relatively understudied, particularly in the United States; however, this group of young people also appears at heightened risk for mental health problems, including anxiety, peer and behavior problems, anger and depression, suicidality, and risk-taking behaviors. It is also known that transgender adults are at increased risk for mental health problems like depression, anxiety, or substance abuse.[9] Fortunately, early appropriate intervention appears to decrease subsequent risk.[10]

As social tolerance increases and LGBT people become more visible, youth may recognize and possibly reveal LGBT feelings or identities in greater numbers and at younger ages.[11,12] As primary care clinicians may encounter these youth, it is important to know how to meet their needs in primary pediatric health settings. Pediatricians who have the first contact also may have an opportunity to recognize and assess any specific mental health needs. Therefore, pediatric clinical competence includes assessing developmental domains of sexuality and gender of all youth, including non-heterosexual orientation, nonconformity in gender expression, and gender-variant identity and any related needs. This includes assessing youths' mental health needs, including their vulnerability and resilience to LGBT-related stigma. As youth may be hesitant to disclose their concerns, it is important that pediatric providers be familiar with and able to intervene appropriately for sexuality, gender-related, and mental health issues.

This article discusses how basic principles of mental health care for LGBT youth can be integrated into routine pediatric care, illustrating ways of doing so with hypothetical case vignettes. In doing so, it assumes basic familiarity with fundamental concepts and skills related to pediatric mental health, and provides clinical guidance in applying mental health practice principles for the LGBT population in pediatric primary care settings.

THE BASICS: LESBIAN, GAY, BISEXUAL, OR TRANSGENDER YOUTH DEVELOPMENT AND MENTAL HEALTH CONCEPTS IN PEDIATRIC PRACTICE
The Pediatrician's Perspective on Development of Sexual Orientation, Gender Expression, and Gender Identity

---

Sexual orientation and gender development: key points for pediatricians

- *Sexual orientation, gender expression, and gender identity* are distinct developmental domains that pediatricians should know and be able to differentiate in youth.

- Forming a sexual orientation and/or a gender identity different from others' expectations and contemplating "coming out" are frequent, unique developmental experiences of LGBT youth.

- A *homosexual* or *bisexual orientation* involves *attraction* to the same sex and can involve emotional and/or erotic feelings, sexual behavior, and/or a youth's identity. These dimensions of sexual orientation may develop over time and may or may not be congruent, sometimes reflecting emotional conflict.

- *Gender expression* refers to gender-related *behavior* in areas such as toy preference, rough-and-tumble play, use of styles, and mannerisms. Some youth display *gender nonconformity*, or variation from group norms, in their expression of gender-related behavior.

- *Gender identity* refers to an individual's personal sense of gender. In some youth it differs from the sex that was recognized and the gender assigned by others at birth. *Gender dysphoria* is distress due to discordance between assigned sex/gender and gender identity, and is distinct from distress due to stigma; each requires appropriate intervention.

- Nonheterosexual orientation, gender nonconformity, and gender dysphoria *can* occur together, but are distinct phenomena and frequently do not occur together. For example, being gay, lesbian or bisexual, sometimes accompanied by a degree of gender nonconformity in youth, is different from being transgender, which may benefit from specific interventions (see Annelou L.C. de Vries' article, "What the Primary Care Pediatrician Needs to Know About Gender Variance in Children and Adolescents," in this issue).

- Each youth can have a distinctive profile of vulnerability and resilience to LGBT-related stress.

Sexual and gender development begins in youth. Gender identity, gender role behavior, and sexual orientation are 3 distinct but interconnected domains of development. In the course of development, youth may exhibit variation from their peers and others' expectations in 1, 2, or all 3 of these domains.[13] Although these may constitute normal variations in development, they may diverge from peer, family, and societal expectations and values, and may elicit negative reactions. Youth who fear being rejected by others may agonize over revealing sexual or gender-related feelings or experiences. This can lead to hiding of (being "in the closet" about) experiences such as same-sex sexual or romantic feelings, nonconformity in gender role behavior, or gender dysphoria, and struggling with revealing these to others ("coming out" to others). These are hallmark concerns that are common among and unique to the development of LGBT youth.

Pediatric clinicians may not be aware that they are caring for an LGBT youth, since some may be not prepared to discuss their sexual and gender development. However, approaching all youth tactfully and confidentially with an awareness that they could be LGBT provides the appropriate guidance, assessment and services if needed. They should monitor how youth are coping with any stresses related to these areas of development, support them, and provide help for any mental health problems that might emerge. In many cases, to preserve the clinical alliance, a clinician may choose to respect a youth's reticence; however, in other situations, an urgent mental health problem may require a pediatric practitioner to take initiative in exploring and addressing an issue.

It is important that pediatric caregivers realize that any youth may be or become lesbian, gay, bisexual or transgender, whether or not they are perceived or have identified themselves as such. Clinicians should be accepting of youth with any expression or disclosure of sexual orientation or gender identity, and foster a clinical relationship characterized by safety and professional support for healthy development, whatever the ultimate sexual orientation or gender identity. They should encourage good peer relations and family connectedness whenever possible, and support resilience and adaptive coping with stress. These principles are well suited to supporting development and providing anticipatory guidance and other well-established models of care.

Sexual Orientation

Human beings differ with regard to their degree of emotional and sexual attraction to those of the opposite or same sex. Most people find that they are predominantly attracted to those of the opposite sex. However, a substantial minority are attracted sexually and emotionally to both or the same sex to a significant or exclusive degree, and thus has a gay, lesbian, or bisexual orientation.[14] These are normal variations in the patterns of human sexual orientation that are frequently first recognized in youth.[15] They may influence the individual's feelings of attraction, patterns of arousal, fantasies, masturbatory or interpersonal sexual behavior, and/or identity. For some, patterns of attraction may change over time, whereas for others they are enduring. Identity may involve a youth's private sense of self, which may be concealed or revealed to others to various degrees over time. These dimensions of sexual orientation may coincide in some individuals, but may not in others.[3]

Most LGB youth gradually discover their sexual orientation over time.[16] As this occurs, some youth struggle with shame, guilt, and the belief that their sexual orientation is unacceptable to themselves and/or others. This may be a source of distress that, in susceptible individuals, may increase the risk of mental health problems. This may be related to negative attitudes or reactions of peers, family, or others in society.[17,18] Many youth with LGB attractions and/or behavior do not have an LGB identity.[19] This may reflect a conflict over sexual orientation in some individuals. It is important that pediatricians monitor for mental health problems that can arise in this context, be aware of their relation to the unique developmental struggles of LGB youth, and intervene appropriately and sensitively.

Gender-Related Behavior and Gender Nonconformity

It is important that pediatric clinicians understand the phenomenon of gender nonconformity. As described in the American Academy of Child and Adolescent Psychiatry

(AACAP) Practice Parameter on LGBT youth,[20] most children display patterns of gender-typed behavior in such areas as toy preferences and degree of inclination toward rough-and-tumble play, dress, mannerisms, or playmate sex preferences; this is *gender-related behavior*. In a given youth, these may approximate group norms to varying degrees. Some youth display patterns that are atypical for their gender, or *gender nonconforming*. Although this can occur to varying degrees, in some youth, nonconformity in gender behavior expression is more significant and/or consistent than in others.[21]

Pediatric clinicians should know that childhood gender nonconformity is sometimes (although not always) associated with nonheterosexual orientation in adolescence.[22] This appears to be especially so for boys, but also sometimes for girls. Although such gender nonconformity is not an illness and not always associated with growing up LGB or T, pediatricians should know about it and its partial association with sexual orientation and gender identity variance, because it can make youth feel different from peers from childhood on and influence how they communicate later with others about their sexual orientation and gender identity.[20] Gender nonconformity also can be a risk factor for adverse phenomena like peer harassment, bullying, and family rejection.[23,24] These problems may place susceptible youth at risk for adverse mental health outcomes like depression, anxiety, and suicidality (see Mark L. Hatzenbuehler and John E. Pachankis' article, "Stigma and Minority Stress as Social Determinants of Health Among LGBT Youth: Research Evidence and Clinical Implications"; Valerie A. Earnshaw and colleagues' article, "LGBT Youth and Bullying"; and Sabra L. Katz-Wise and colleagues' article, "LGBT Youth and Family Acceptance," in this issue). Fortunately, pediatric clinicians can intervene in ways described in these articles to decrease their likelihood.

Gender Identity and Gender Dysphoria

Pediatricians should understand *gender identity* and *gender dysphoria*, a unique phenomena that may benefit from specific pediatric interventions. In contrast with gender-related behavior, *gender* refers to a person's social (and usually legal) assignment as female or male in a society with a binary gender system, or as female, male, or an alternate category in a society that has them (for example, India recently established legal recognition of *hijras*). Gender is usually recognized at birth based on the appearance of the external genitalia corresponding with the genetic makeup and its phenotypic expression. *Gender identity* refers to an individual's sense of gender. Some youth discover that their gender identity is different from the one assigned, or that they are between genders, identify with both genders, feel gender neutral, are "gender queer," or "expansive" – terms meaning not conventionally categorizable that are used with increasing frequency by youth diagnosed with gender dysphoria.[25,26]

Gender identity and gender expression are different. Gender dysphoria frequently occurs in conjunction with marked behavioral gender nonconformity, but also can occur without gender-nonconforming behavior in some people. In contrast with gender nonconformity alone, gender dysphoria can benefit from specific interventions (see Annelou L.C. de Vries and colleagues' article, "What the Primary Care Pediatrician Needs to Know About Gender Variance in Children and Adolescents," in this issue). The *Diagnostic and Statistical Manual of Mental Disorders, 5th Edition* (DSM-5)[27] defines gender dysphoria as distress about a *gender identity* that differs from the individual's socially assigned sex/gender. By definition, gender dysphoria is distress about the discordance between a youth's gender identity and sex assigned at birth. However, stigma, sometimes enacted as harassment, bullying, or family rejection, can be another important source of distress.[28]

Clinical samples with limited follow-up have found prepubertal gender dysphoria to be transient in some youth and persistent in others.[22,29–31] Predictors of persistence in clinical cohorts include a greater intensity of gender dysphoria and meeting criteria for a DSM diagnosis; a cognitive or affective cross-gender identification (that is, saying "I am" or "I feel like" rather than "I wish I were the other sex"); having a younger age of presentation; being a birth assigned male; and having gone through an early social role transition (especially in birth assigned boys).[29,30]

When gender dysphoria is present in adolescence, it usually remains a stable trait. Although adolescents can grow up to have any sexual orientation, studies limited to specialty clinic cohorts have found children diagnosed with gender dysphoria to develop nonheterosexual orientations more frequently than most children.[22,30–33] Further research, including population samples and long-term follow-up studies, is needed to determine how these findings apply to youth seen by general pediatricians and to guide best practices.

Distinguishing Gender Nonconformity and Gender Dysphoria

A youth's feelings of gender dysphoria may first come to a primary care clinician's attention in a variety of ways. These may include issues or concerns raised directly by the youth, parents, or others. It is important that clinicians understand that gender-nonconforming behavior and gender dysphoria are different, albeit sometimes co-occurring, phenomena.[34] In some youth, gender dysphoria may be suggested by significant, persistent gender-nonconforming behavior, whereas in others, gender-nonconforming behavior occurs without gender dysphoria. Distinguishing youth with gender-nonconforming behavior alone from those who may be experiencing gender dysphoria can be clinically challenging; for example, in youth not yet ready or developmentally able to verbalize their thoughts and feelings, who have comorbid mental health issues that interfere with doing so, or who are experiencing uncertainty about their identity for other reasons. Nevertheless, making this distinction is important, because youth diagnosed with gender dysphoria may benefit from gender treatments (see Annelou L.C. de Vries and colleagues' article, "What the Primary Care Pediatrician Needs to Know About Gender Variance in Children and Adolescents," in this issue). However, not all behaviorally gender-nonconforming youth experience gender dysphoria. Many or most gender-nonconforming youth who pediatricians may see will not experience gender dysphoria, including many nontransgender youth growing up gay, lesbian, or bisexual. In contrast to transgender youth, some nontransgender gay, lesbian, or bisexual youth may fear being regarded as not belonging to their assigned birth gender.[34] For them, gender-affirming care would not involve the same treatments described for those diagnosed with gender dysphoria described in Annelou L.C. de Vries and colleagues' article, "What the Primary Care Pediatrician Needs to Know About Gender Variance in Children and Adolescents," in this issue.

To assist with accurate assessment and appropriate interventions, pediatric clinicians may find it helpful to obtain consultation from developmental or mental health specialists with clinical competence in sexual orientation and gender. These may be available locally, by consulting published guidelines and tools for assessment,[20,34,35] or through national organizations such as the AACAP (www.aacap.org), the National LGBT Health Education Center (www.lgbthealtheducation.org), the Substance Abuse and Mental Health Services Administration (SAMHSA)'s National Suicide Resources (www.suicidepreventionlifeline.org), The Trevor Project (www.thetrevorproject.org/pages/get-help-now#tc), or the Crisis Text Line (www.crisistextline.org/textline/). It is important for pediatric care providers to allow children and adolescents to discover and reveal themselves over time, to consider both immediate and long-term needs in the context of current research, to promote well-being and avoid harm, and resist premature conclusions about anyone's future developmental endpoints.

MEETING MENTAL HEALTH NEEDS OF LESBIAN, GAY, BISEXUAL, OR TRANSGENDER YOUTH IN PEDIATRIC PRACTICE

Key competencies in LGBT mental health practice for pediatric providers are as follows:

- Be familiar with key mental health guidelines, community resources, and the continuum of mental health intervention for all (not just LGBT) youth.
- For LGBT youth, know AACAP's mental health practice principles (listed in next section).
- Be able to integrate LGBT-specific mental health principles into pediatric practice.
- Know how to apply these principles in the context of youth, family and cultural values, community resources, and practice setting.

Basic principles of mental health care in pediatric settings, including principles of screening, assessment, intervention, and referral for providers of pediatric care, are outlined in basic texts[36] and are available through national organizations like the American Academy of Pediatrics' www.healthychildren.org site's material on Mental Health Initiatives, as well as AACAP (www.aacap.org). These general principles of mental health care are relevant to LGBT youth as well. In addition to these universal principles, as a special population, LGBT youth have unique mental health needs that warrant special principles of pediatric practice.[20,37] Given the important role that pediatric clinicians play in safeguarding their patients' healthy development including their mental health and the elevated risk for problems in LGBT youth, being able to adapt principles of mental health care for LGBT youth to pediatric settings is an important aspect of clinical competence.

Pediatric care settings vary widely, ranging from primary settings, such as school nurse offices, primary care clinics, and pediatric offices, to urgent care settings, such as emergency rooms, and specialized settings, such as academic tertiary care centers. These may be located in a range of communities, from urban to suburban to rural, with an equally wide range of mental health resources, sociocultural contexts, and community norms. Clinical encounters also may vary in duration, intensity, and type, because pediatric care is often well-child care or focused on immediate clinical needs. The mental health interventions that can be integrated into this array of settings vary widely in level of service and degree of structure, and may include anticipatory guidance, screening, specialized referral, consultation, integrated and collaborative care, outpatient treatment or inpatient treatment, and specialized emergency and crisis services. Obviously, the mental health services offered will vary by treatment setting, model of care, and resources. An understanding of youths' mental health needs can help clinical leadership to best organize available resources to meet those needs, including for LGBT youth.

When clinical questions emerge about sexual orientation and gender development, it is important that pediatricians understand the youth and family, and what the questions mean in the context of their individual and shared values, culture, and community. They should remain alert to common mental health problems with significant morbidity and mortality, such as depression, substance use, and suicidality, and deal with mental health emergencies appropriately, as these may entail serious risks of morbidity and mortality. They should know sources of distress in LGBT youths' lives, such as community stigma, bullying, and family nonacceptance; understand the individual's vulnerabilities and strengths; and be able to identify sources of coping, such as individual resilience and sources of interpersonal and community support. They should be familiar with local mental health, family support, and community resources (for a partial listing see the appendix at the end of this volume) and be ready to intervene with mental health interventions, such as referral, consultation, or treatment based on the individual's needs and within the practice model and resources.

Some LGBT youth are at increased risk for substance abuse (see Romulo Aromin Jr's article, "Substance Abuse Prevention, Assessment and Treatment for LGBT Youth," in this issue) or disordered eating (see Zachary McClain and Rebecka Peebles' article, "Body Image and Disordered Eating Among LGBT Youth," in this issue), especially those with body image dissatisfaction related to gender nonconformity or gender dysphoria. Certain LGBT youth may require child protective or social services in addition to mental health intervention. For example, LGBT youth who become socially or economically marginalized or homeless following rejection by families may be at increased risk for behavior like unprotected sex.[38]

Mental Health Screening for Lesbian, Gay, Bisexual, or Transgender Youth in Pediatric Practice

Early identification of significant mental health problems and prompt referral and treatment are essential. Some form of systematic screening for mental health problems can be a useful component of pediatric care. This might be done by routine interview in the context of a clinical relationship. It might also employ one or a number of screening instruments, often a paper-and-pencil questionnaire completed by youth, their caregivers, and/or school personnel, that can help identify symptoms of mental health problems.[2] When using a screening instrument for LGBT youth, it is important to know whether it was specifically designed and standardized for use in this population, and whether it includes appropriate questions pertinent to issues like sexual orientation, gender identity, and gender role behaviors, or stigmatizing experiences, such as family nonacceptance or bullying. For youth who conceal LGBT feelings, behaviors, or identities, it is important to consider whether nondisclosure impairs an instrument's clinical reliability and validity. More research is needed on the best way to screen specifically LGBT youth for mental health problems.

Apart from structured instruments, sound clinical judgment and interviewing skills remain indispensable parts of screening. A thoughtful clinical interview can be key in ascertaining whether a child or adolescent is experiencing significant emotional, behavioral, or other mental health problems. Sometimes this information can be obtained directly from the youth and, if appropriate, from caregivers. However, confidentiality is a special consideration in the treatment of LGBT youth and in adolescent sexual and reproductive health generally (see Scott E. Hadland and colleagues' article "Caring for LGBTQ Youth in Inclusive and Affirmative Environments," in this issue). It is important to use sound clinical judgment in preserving confidentiality, to not undermine the clinical alliance, to know local confidentiality guidelines pertaining to special health care topics like sexual and mental health, and to integrate these in care.

Applying Principles of Mental Health Practice with Lesbian, Gay, Bisexual, or Transgender Youth in Pediatric Practice

The following is a summary of practice principles reprinted from the AACAP's Practice Parameter on LGBT Youth,[20] which is available through AACAP's website (www.aacap.org) and discussed in webinars and related material available through the National LGBT Health Education Center (www.lgbthealtheducation.org). The application of these principles is illustrated in 2 composite, hypothetical vignettes that follow (**Box 1**). The following hypothetical case vignettes illustrate the benefit of mental health intervention by a pediatrician. They emphasize the importance of the clinical principles described previously. These include the need for special consideration of issues of psychosexual assessment, confidentiality, family dynamics and values, psychiatric risk factors, support of healthy development, understanding of general principles of sexual orientation and gender identity development, the ability to use appropriate clinical liaison, and the use of community resources.

CASE 1: A FEMALE TO MALE TRANSGENDER ADOLESCENT WITH FAMILY NONACCEPTANCE, DEPRESSION, ANXIETY, AND SUICIDE ATTEMPTS

A Hispanic patient with an assigned female birth gender, an only child in a low-income, urban immigrant family, had depression, anxiety, suicidality, family arguments, and school difficulty starting at age 12 around puberty. The patient displayed marked gender nonconformity, preferring stereotypically masculine clothing and

---

Box 1
Practice principles outlined in the American Academy of Child and Adolescent Psychiatry's practice parameter on lesbian, gay, bisexual, and transgender youth

"Principle 1. A comprehensive diagnostic evaluation should include an age-appropriate assessment of psychosexual development for all youths.

Principle 2. The need for confidentiality in the clinical alliance is a special consideration in the assessment of sexual and gender minority youth.

Principle 3. Family dynamics pertinent to sexual orientation, gender nonconformity, and gender identity should be explored in the context of the cultural values of the youth, family, and community.

Principle 4. Clinicians should inquire about circumstances commonly encountered by youth with sexual and gender minority status that confer increased psychiatric risk.

Principle 5. Clinicians should aim to foster healthy psychosexual development in sexual and gender minority youth and protect the individual's full capacity for integrated identity formation and adaptive functioning.

Principle 6. Clinicians should be aware that there is no evidence that sexual orientation can be altered through therapy, and that attempts to do so may be harmful.

Principle 7. Clinicians should be aware of current evidence on the natural course of gender discordance and associated psychopathology in children and adolescents in choosing the treatment goals and modality.

Principle 8. Clinicians should be prepared to consult and act as a liaison with schools, community agencies, and other health care providers, advocating for the unique needs of sexual and gender minority youth and their families.

Principle 9. Mental health professionals should be aware of community and professional resources relevant to sexual and gender minority youth.

From Adelson SL, American Academy of Child and Adolescent Psychiatry (AACAP) Committee on Quality Issues (CQI). Practice parameter on gay, lesbian or bisexual sexual orientation, gender-nonconformity, and gender discordance in children and adolescents. J Am Acad Child Adolesc Psychiatry 2012;51(9):957–74; with permission.

hairstyles. At age 13, the patient was referred to pediatric endocrinologists for obesity and hirsutism, and also to a child and adolescent psychiatrist for suicidal ideation following a verbal argument with the patient's parents. The patient's parents, who speak only Spanish and felt isolated in their community without extended family support, feared being further stigmatized by the patient's gender nonconformity, attributed it to a deviant peer group and popular American media influences, and severely criticized and tried to limit it. Child Protective Services had to intervene when the patient attempted to join an LGBT youth group to decrease social isolation and the father became physically abusive. The patient attempted suicide twice. The mental health treatment team diagnosed major depressive disorder, recurrent type, panic disorder, and, although the patient had never disclosed it to the pediatrician or endocrinologist, gender dysphoria. After the second suicide attempt at age 15, the patient identified the source of anguish as gender dysphoria and fear of rejection for it. The patient discussed this with peers, but did not disclose it to any adults until opening up to the therapist. The patient disclosed his male gender identity to his parents with the support of his mental health treatment team at age 15. Through the support of his therapist, he was able to engage his mother in a process to better understand his experience. His father has refused to be involved in his care. The patient was initially treated within a psychodynamic psychotherapy framework, but when he started engaging in self-injurious behaviors, the model changed to dialectical behavior therapy. He has benefited from his treatment with an improvement in his mood and anxiety, but family work continues to address ongoing ambivalent acceptance.

CASE 2: A LESBIAN FEMALE ADOLESCENT WITH TRUANCY, RUNNING AWAY, MULTIPLE SEXUALLY TRANSMITTED INFECTIONS, AND HIGH-RISK SEXUAL BEHAVIOR

The patient is an African American female individual from a northeastern US city who was referred for a psychiatric assessment at age 15 after her medical provider became concerned about recurrent STIs. She stated that, after she revealed same-sex attractions and a lesbian identity to her mother, her mother's boyfriend sexually molested her to thwart her same-sex attractions. Child Protective Services was notified, but the patient later retracted her story, and the charges were unsubstantiated. Her mother did not want her back, blaming her for creating trouble, and sent her to live with her grandmother in the South. She eventually moved back to the Northeast and initially stayed with friends, but eventually became homeless and involved with alcohol, marijuana, and cocaine. She used social media to hook up and trade heterosexual sex with males for money. At age 17, she was arrested and entered the foster care system, but eloped from every family placement and eventually entered a group home for teens. She was marginally engaged in outpatient mental health care and had the Diagnoses of posttraumatic stress disorder, major depressive disorder, and cannabis abuse. She denied that she had been victimized or traumatized, and remained guarded, isolated, and withdrawn. However, on entering a group therapy treatment, she connected with LGBT peers, slowly disclosed her trauma, and began a therapeutic process using trauma-focused cognitive behavior therapy. She struggled with the betrayal of her mother and trusting others, but formed prosocial relationships with her therapy group and developed a sense of community with other sexual minority youth. She has benefited from group interventions and peer support so as to decrease high-risk behavior, remain in her group home, and participate in a high school equivalency program.

REFERENCES

1. Centers for Disease Control and Prevention. 10 leading causes of death by age group, United States-2012. 2014. Available at: http://www.cdc.gov/injury/wisqars/. Accessed January 25, 2015.
2. Walter H, DeMaso M. Assessment and interviewing. In: Kliegman RM, Stanton BF, St Geme J, et al, editors. Nelson textbook of pediatrics. 20th edition. Philadelphia: Elsevier; 2015. p. 124–7.
3. Adelson SL, Schuster MA. Gay, lesbian & bisexual adolescents. In: Kliegman RM, Stanton BF, Geme JSt, et al, editors. Nelson textbook of pediatrics. 20th edition. Philadelphia: Elsevier; 2015. p. 934–7.
4. Agency for Healthcare Research and Quality. Mental disorders among most costly conditions in children. AHRQ News and Numbers. 2009. Available at: http://www.ahrq.gov/news/nn/nn042209.htm. Accessed January 17, 2013.
5. Coker TR, Austin SB, Schuster MA. The health and health care of lesbian, gay, and bisexual adolescents. Annu Rev Public Health 2010;31:457–77.
6. Makadon HJ, Mayer KH, Potter J, et al, editors. The Fenway guide to lesbian, gay, bisexual and transgender health. 2nd edition. Washington, DC: American College of Physicians; 2015.
7. Mustanski BS, Garofalo R, Emerson EM. Mental health disorders, psychological distress, and suicidality in a diverse sample of lesbian, gay, bisexual, and transgender youths. Am J Public Health 2010;100(12):2426–32.
8. Liu RT, Mustanski B. Suicidal ideation and self-harm in lesbian, gay, bisexual, and transgender youth. Am J Prev Med 2012;42:221–8.
9. Institute of Medicine (US), Committee on Lesbian, Gay, Bisexual, and Transgender Health Issues and Research Gaps and Opportunities. The health of lesbian, gay, bisexual, and transgender people: building a foundation for better understanding. Washington, DC: National Academies Press (US); 2011.
10. de Vries AL, Steensma TD, Doreleijers TA, et al. Puberty suppression in adolescents with gender identity disorder: a prospective follow-up study. J Sex Med 2010;8:2276–83.
11. de Vries AL, Cohen-Kettenis PT. Clinical management of gender dysphoria in children and adolescents: the Dutch approach. J Homosex 2012;59(3):301–20.
12. Wood H, Sasaki S, Bradley SJ, et al. Patterns of referral to a gender identity service for children and adolescents (1976–2011): age, sex ratio, and sexual orientation. J Sex Marital Ther 2013;39:1–6.
13. Rosario M, Schrimshaw EW. The sexual identity development and health of lesbian, gay, and bisexual adolescents: an ecological perspective. In: Patterson CJ, D'Augelli AR, editors. Handbook of psychology and sexual orientation. New York: Oxford; 2013. p. 87–101.
14. Mustanski B, Birkett M, Greene GJ, et al. The association between sexual orientation identity and behavior varies across race/ethnicity, gender, and age in a probability sample of high school students. Am J Public Health 2014;104:237–44.
15. Rosario M, Schrimshaw EW. Theories and etiologies of sexual orientation. In: Tolman DL, Diamond LM, editors. APA handbook of sexuality and psychology, vol. 1. Washington, DC: American Psychological Association; 2014. p. 555–96.
16. Remafedi G, Resnick M, Blum R, et al. Demography of sexual orientation in adolescents. Pediatrics 1992;89:714–21.
17. Hatzenbuehler ML. The social environment and suicide attempts in lesbian, gay, and bisexual youth. Pediatrics 2011;127(5):896–903.

18. Meyer IH. Prejudice, social stress, and mental health in lesbian, gay, and bisexual populations: conceptual issues and research evidence. Psychol Bull 2003; 129(5):674–97.

19. Kann L, Olsen EO, McManus T, et al, Centers for Disease Control and Prevention (CDC). Sexual identity, sex of sexual contacts, and health-risk behaviors among students in grades 9-12–youth risk behavior surveillance, selected sites, United States, 2001-2009. MMWR Surveill Summ 2011;60(7):1–133.

20. Adelson SL, American Academy of Child and Adolescent Psychiatry (AACAP) Committee on Quality Issues (CQI). Practice parameter on gay, lesbian or bisexual sexual orientation, gender-nonconformity, and gender discordance in children and adolescents. J Am Acad Child Adolesc Psychiatry 2012;51(9): 957–74.

21. Ruble DN, Martin CL, Berenbaum SA. Gender development. In: Damon W, Lerner RM, editors. Handbook of child psychology. 6th edition. Hoboken (NJ): Wiley InterScience; 2007. p. 858–932 [electronic resource].

22. Bailey JM, Zucker KJ. Childhood sex-typed behavior and sexual orientation: a conceptual analysis and quantitative review. Dev Psychol 1995;31(1):43–55.

23. Roberts AL, Rosario M, Slopen N, et al. Childhood gender nonconformity, bullying victimization, and depressive symptoms across adolescence and early adulthood: an 11-year longitudinal study. J Am Acad Child Adolesc Psychiatry 2013;52(2):143–52.

24. Ryan C, Huebner D, Diaz RM, et al. Family rejection as a predictor of negative health outcomes in white and Latino lesbian, gay, and bisexual young adults. Pediatrics 2009;123(1):346–52.

25. Kuper LE, Nussbaum R, Mustanski B. Exploring the diversity of gender and sexual orientation identities in an online sample of transgender individuals. J Sex Res 2012;49(2-3):244–54.

26. Harrison J, Grant J, Herman JL. A gender not listed here: Genderqueers, gender rebels, and otherwise in the National Transgender Discrimination Survey; 2012.

27. American Psychiatric Association. Diagnostic and statistical manual of mental disorders. 5th edition. Washington, DC: American Psychiatric Publishing; 2013.

28. Nuttbrock L, Hwahng S, Bockting W, et al. Psychiatric impact of gender-related abuse across the life course of male-to-female transgender persons. J Sex Res 2010;47(1):12–23.

29. Steensma TD, McGuire JK, Kreukels BP, et al. Factors associated with desistence and persistence of childhood gender dysphoria: a quantitative follow-up study. J Am Acad Child Adolesc Psychiatry 2013;52:582–90.

30. Wallien MS, Cohen-Kettenis PT. Psychosexual outcome of gender-dysphoric children. J Am Acad Child Adolesc Psychiatry 2008;47(12):1413–23.

31. Drummond KD, Bradley SJ, Peterson-Badali M, et al. A follow-up study of girls with gender identity disorder. Dev Psychol 2008;44(1):34–45.

32. Green R. The Sissy-Boy Syndrome and the Development of Homosexuality. New Haven: Yale University Press; 1987.

33. Steensma TD, Biemond R, de Boer F, et al. Desisting and persisting gender dysphoria after childhood: a qualitative follow-up study. Clin Child Psychol Psychiatry 2011;16(4):499–516.

34. Leibowitz S, Adelson S, Telingator C. Gender nonconformity and gender discordance in childhood and adolescence: developmental considerations and the clinical approach. In: Makadon HJ, Mayer KH, Potter J, et al, editors. The Fenway guide to lesbian, gay, bisexual and transgender health. 2nd edition. Washington, DC: American College of Physicians; 2015. p. 421–58.

35. Bockting WO. Sexual identity development. In: Kliegman RM, Stanton BF, Geme JSt, et al, editors. Nelson textbook of pediatrics. 20th edition. Philadelphia: Elsevier; 2015. p. 931–4.
36. Kliegman RM, Stanton BF, St Geme J, et al, editors. Nelson textbook of pediatrics. 20th edition. Philadelphia: Elsevier; 2015.
37. Makadon HJ, Mayer KH, Potter J, et al. The Fenway Guide to Lesbian, Gay, Bisexual and Transgender Health. 2nd Edition. American College of Physicians; 2015.
38. Marshall BD, Shannon K, Kerr T, et al. Survival sex work and increased HIV risk among sexual minority street-involved youth. J Acquir Immune Defic Syndr 2010;53(5):661–4.

Stigma and Minority Stress as Social Determinants of Health Among Lesbian, Gay, Bisexual, and Transgender Youth

CrossMark

Research Evidence and Clinical Implications

Mark L. Hatzenbuehler, PhD[a],*, John E. Pachankis, PhD[b]

KEYWORDS

- Stigma • Minority stress • Health • LGBT youth

KEY POINTS

- Stigma occurs at multiple levels to affect the health of lesbian, gay, bisexual, and transgender (LGBT) youth, including structural, interpersonal, and individual levels.
- Stigma disrupts cognitive (eg, vigilance), affective (eg, rumination), interpersonal (eg, isolation), and physiologic (eg, stress reactivity) processes that influence the health of LGBT youth.
- These stigma-inducing mechanisms can be targeted with both clinical and public health interventions to reduce LGBT health disparities among youth.
- Multicomponent interventions are likely to be most effective in reducing the negative health consequences of exposure to stigma among this population.

The other articles in this issue review the literature documenting health disparities related to sexual orientation and gender identity among youth. Relative to their heterosexual and cis-gender peers, lesbian, gay, bisexual, and transgender (LGBT) youth are at increased risk for adverse mental health outcomes (eg, depression, anxiety, and suicidality; see Stewart L. Adelson and colleagues' article, "Development and Mental Health of LGBT Youth in Pediatric Practice," in this issue), substance use (see Romulo Alcalde Aromin Jr's article, "Substance Abuse Prevention, Assessment & Treatment for LGBT Youth," in this issue), human immunodeficiency virus (HIV)

Disclosure Statement: The authors have nothing to disclose. This article was funded, in part, by a Mentored Research Scientist Development Award to M.L. Hatzenbuehler (DA032558).

[a] Department of Sociomedical Sciences, Mailman School of Public Health, Columbia University, 722 West 168th Street, Room 549B, New York, NY 10032, USA; [b] Chronic Disease Epidemiology: Social & Behavioral Sciences, Yale School of Public Health, 60 College Street, Suite 316, New Haven, CT 06510, USA

* Corresponding author.

E-mail address: mlh2101@cumc.columbia.edu

infection and other sexually transmitted infections (see Sarah M. Wood and colleagues' article, "HIV, Other Sexually Transmitted Infections, and Sexual Health in LGBT Youth," in this issue), and disordered eating (see Zachary McClain and Rebecka Peebles's article, "Body Image and Disordered Eating Among LGBT Youth," in this issue). Having established the existence of LGBT health disparities among youth, the field has turned to the identification of factors that can explain them.[1]

In this article, we review theories and evidence for stigma and minority stress as determinants of LGBT health disparities among youth. We begin by briefly reviewing theories of stigma and minority stress. Next, we cover empirical evidence bearing on the role that stigma at individual, interpersonal, and structural levels plays in conferring risk for negative health outcomes among LGBT youth. We then cover the myriad processes that are disrupted by stigma—ranging from cognitive (eg, sensitivity to rejection), affective (eg, emotional response), interpersonal (eg, social relationships), and physiologic (eg, reactivity to stress)—that in turn contribute to poor health among this population. Finally, we review emerging evidence for clinical and public health interventions aimed at reducing LGBT health disparities among youth and conclude with a discussion of future directions for research and interventions.

THEORIES OF STIGMA AND MINORITY STRESS

Link and Phelan[2] (2001) put forward a widely used conceptualization of stigma that recognized the overlap in meaning among concepts like stigma, labeling, stereotyping, and discrimination. Their conceptualization defines stigma as the co-occurrence of several interrelated components:

> In the first component, people distinguish and label human differences. In the second, dominant cultural beliefs link labeled persons to undesirable characteristics – to negative stereotypes. In the third, labeled persons are placed in distinct categories so as to accomplish some degree of separation of "us" from "them." In the fourth, labeled persons experience status loss and discrimination that lead to unequal outcomes. Stigmatization is entirely contingent on access to social, economic and political power that allows the identification of differentness, the construction of stereotypes, the separation of labeled persons into distinct categories and the full execution of disapproval, rejection, exclusion and discrimination. Thus, we apply the term stigma when elements of labeling, stereotyping, separation, status loss and discrimination co-occur in a power situation that allows them to unfold.[2]

Drawing on insights from the stigma literature, Meyer (2003) developed the minority stress theory, which refers to the "excess stress to which individuals from stigmatized social categories are exposed as a result of their social, often a minority, position."[3] Meyer (2003) conceptualized these stressors as unique (in that they are additive to general stressors that are experienced by all people and therefore require adaptations above and beyond those required of the nonstigmatized), chronic (in that they are related to relatively stable social structures such as laws and social policies), and socially based (in that they stem from social/structural forces rather than individual events or conditions).[3] Minority stress theory therefore posits that health disparities observed in LGBT populations do not reflect psychological issues inherent to LGBT individuals, but rather are the end result of persistent stigma directed toward them.[3] Originally developed to explain sexual orientation disparities in mental health, the theory has recently been applied to physical health disparities[4] and to understanding health disparities related to gender identity.[5,6]

STIGMA AND MINORITY STRESS AS RISK INDICATORS FOR ADVERSE HEALTH OUTCOMES AMONG LESBIAN, GAY, BISEXUAL, AND TRANSGENDER YOUTH

It has long been recognized that stigma and minority stress exist at individual, interpersonal, and structural levels (**Fig. 1**). In the following section, we selectively review research evidence bearing on the health consequences of stigma across these levels for LGBT youth.

Individual

Individual forms of stigma refer to individuals' cognitive, affective, and behavioral responses to stigma. In this section, we focus on 3 individual-level stigma processes that have received the most empirical attention with LGBT populations: internalized homophobia/transphobia, rejection sensitivity, and concealment.

Internalized homophobia/transphobia refers to the internalization of negative societal attitudes about one's sexual orientation or gender identity. Such negative self-regard has been associated with poor health outcomes among LGBT individuals. For example, sexual minority adults' experiences with internalized homophobia are positively associated with alcohol and drug use,[7] HIV risk behaviors,[8] and bulimic behavior.[9] Internalized homophobia among sexual minority male youth is associated prospectively with sexual risk behavior.[10] In addition, internalized transphobia is associated with increased risk of lifetime suicide attempts among transgender adults.[11] Thus, experiences with internalized homophobia and transphobia can arouse negative feelings about one's own social group, which have been linked to unhealthy behaviors that put LGBT individuals at risk for health problems.

Experiences with stigma and minority stress also make targets sensitive to rejection. Stigma-based rejection sensitivity describes the psychological process through which some individuals learn to anxiously anticipate rejection because of previous experiences with prejudice and discrimination toward their group membership.[12] Sensitivity to possible rejection becomes particularly salient during adolescence,[13] and rejection during this time predicts mental health problems across the lifespan.[14] Adolescents who become aware of a stigmatized personal status during this developmental period

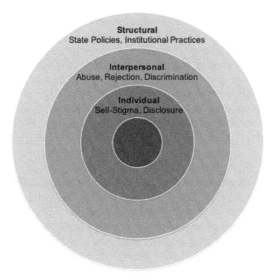

Fig. 1. Stigma as a multilevel construct.

and who are particularly sensitive to rejection of their stigma may be particularly likely to develop unhealthy coping strategies to fend off expected rejection in potentially threatening contexts.[15] Most studies on rejection sensitivity among LGBT populations have been conducted with adult samples,[16] but recent studies have shown that young gay and bisexual men high in rejection sensitivity use condoms less often, which is mediated by their diminished condom use self-efficacy.[17] Although rejection sensitivity should also affect the health of LGBT youth, this has not yet been documented empirically.

Experiences with sexual orientation-related stigma can lead sexual and gender minority individuals to engage in concealment behaviors, which refers to hiding their identity to avoid future victimization.[18] Although this can serve as a positive coping strategy in the short term by helping sexual minorities to avoid victimization,[19] it is associated with a host of psychological consequences in the long term, including depressive symptoms,[20] negative affect and anxiety,[21] poor self-esteem and elevated psychiatric symptoms,[22] and psychological strain.[23] Concealment can also harm sexual minority physical health by affecting the care they receive from medical professionals. For example, sexual minority adults have special medical needs that likely go unmet if they conceal their sexual orientation from health care workers.[24,25] Transgender individuals who cannot or choose not to access gender affirmation procedures, and those who transition later in life after already having developed secondary sex characteristics, may be at increased risk of stigma given their visible gender nonconformity.[6,26] In fact, the degree to which others can tell whether an individual is transgender has been linked to discrimination and poor mental and physical health outcomes.[27] Delaying the transition process while concealing one's transgender identity may contribute to psychological distress in adolescents and adults.[28] Concealment by those who have not transitioned can restrict access to transition-related medical services, whereas concealment by those who have transitioned can lead to inappropriate medical care for relevant anatomy.[29,30]

Interpersonal

Interpersonal forms of stigma refer to prejudice and discrimination as expressed by one person toward another—that is, to interactional processes that occur between the stigmatized and the nonstigmatized. Interpersonal stigma not only includes intentional, overt actions, such as bias-based hate crimes,[31] but also unintentional, covert actions, like microaggressions.[32] Research on interpersonal forms of stigma among LGBT youth has tended to focus on 2 forms: peer victimization and bullying (see Valerie A. Earnshaw and colleagues' article, "LGBT Youth and Bullying," in this issue) and parental abuse and rejection (see Sabra L. Katz-Wise and colleagues' article, "LGBT Youth and Family Acceptance," in this issue). Given that these 2 topics are covered in greater detail in other articles in this issue, we will not discuss them here.

Structural

Structural forms of stigma refer to stigma processes that occur above the individual and interpersonal levels of analyses and are defined as "societal-level conditions, cultural norms, and institutional policies that constrain the opportunities, resources, and wellbeing of the stigmatized."[33] Compared with research on individual and interpersonal forms of stigma, there has been less empirical work on stigma at the structural level. Nevertheless, an emerging body of evidence highlights the role that structural stigma plays in the production of LGBT health inequalities (for a review, see Hatzenbuehler[34]). We review several illustrative examples of this research in the following section.

Studies of structural stigma and the health of LGBT youth have followed 2 broad approaches. In the first approach, researchers examine the association between a single indicator of structural stigma and health outcomes among LGBT populations. In an example of this work, researchers obtained data on neighborhood-level LGBT hate crimes involving assaults or assaults with battery from the Boston Police Department that were linked to individual-level data on health and sexual orientation from a population-based sample of Boston adolescents. Sexual minority youth residing in neighborhoods with higher rates of LGBT assault-based hate crimes were significantly more likely to report adverse health outcomes, including suicidal ideation and suicide attempts,[35] bullying,[36] and marijuana use,[37] than were sexual minority youth residing in neighborhoods with lower LGBT assault-based hate crime rates. No associations between LGBT assault-based hate crimes and these adverse health outcomes were found among heterosexual adolescents, indicating that the results were specific to sexual minority respondents. Further, no relationships were observed between overall neighborhood-level violent crimes and these adverse health outcomes among sexual minority adolescents, which provided evidence for the specificity of the results to LGBT assault-based hate crimes.

In the second methodological approach, researchers create a composite index of structural stigma that includes multiple components (rather than examining single indicators of structural stigma), and then examine whether this index predicts adverse health outcomes among LGBT youth. For instance, Hatzenbuehler[38] (2011) created an index of structural stigma surrounding sexual minorities that included 4 different components: density of same-sex couples, proportion of gay–straight alliances per public high school, 5 policies related to sexual orientation discrimination (eg, same-sex marriage laws, antidiscrimination statutes), and aggregated public opinion toward homosexuality.[38] Several studies have shown that this composite variable of structural stigma is associated with adverse health outcomes among LGBT youth. In 1 cross-sectional study, the risk of attempting suicide in the past 12 months was 20% greater among LGB youth living in counties with higher levels of structural stigma compared with those living in counties with lower levels of structural stigma.[38] In longitudinal studies, researchers have shown that sexual minority youth living in low structural stigma states are less likely to smoke over time than sexual minority youth in high structural stigma states[39]; moreover, sexual orientation disparities in marijuana use and other illicit drug use are significantly smaller in low structural stigma states than in high structural stigma states.[40]

STIGMA-INDUCING MECHANISMS

Thus far, we have discussed research establishing that stigma and minority stress confer risk for a variety of adverse health outcomes among LGBT youth. An obvious question arises: How is it that stigma and minority stress "get under the skin" to contribute to poor health? The identification of mechanisms linking stigma to health is important because it points to potential targets for both clinical and public health interventions aimed at reducing LGBT health disparities. In this section, we selectively review research on several psychosocial (cognitive, affective, and interpersonal) and physiologic mechanisms through which stigma and minority stress impair the health of LGBT youth (for more comprehensive reviews on this topic, see[4,41,42]).

Vigilance

Experiences with stigma and minority stressors can alter cognitive processes in ways that impact health.[41] A substantial body of research has shown that experiences with stigma make minority individuals vigilant of their social environment to anticipate and avoid stigmatizing encounters.[43] Studies in the general population have supported a link between perceptual vigilance and cardiovascular functioning, demonstrating heightened systolic and diastolic blood pressure among participants who were vigilant to negative social messages.[44] Further, experiences with stigma make sexual minority individuals vigilant to threats in their social environment,[45] which in turn is associated with adverse mental health outcomes, such as depressive symptoms.[8]

Rumination

Emotion regulation is defined as the "conscious and nonconscious strategies [people] use to increase, maintain, or decrease one or more components of an emotional response."[46] Repeated encounters with stigma and minority stressors may lead LGB individuals to ruminate, which is a maladaptive emotion regulation strategy characterized by repeated focus on the causes and symptoms of distress.[47] Prospective studies have revealed that individuals with a high degree of life stress develop increasingly ruminative tendencies.[48] Specific to sexual minority populations, Hatzenbuehler and colleagues[49] have found that LGB adolescents and adults tend to ruminate more than their heterosexual counterparts. Further, ruminative tendencies have been specifically linked to minority stress in particular. Sexual minority young adults were especially likely to ruminate on days when they encountered stigma-related stressors related to their sexual orientation, and such rumination was associated with psychological distress.[50]

Loneliness

Stigma and minority stressors may increase feelings of loneliness among LGBT individuals, which in turn can affect interpersonal relationships. Loneliness is common among members of stigmatized groups,[51] and it may be especially so for sexual and gender minorities, who frequently encounter rejection from family members and friends.[52] In addition, fears of future rejection and negative evaluation lead individuals with concealable stigmas (eg, homosexuality) to avoid entering into close relationships for fear of others' discovering their stigma, which over time leads to more loneliness, introversion, psychological distress, and social anxiety.[53]

Physiologic Mechanisms Related to Stress Response

Finally, physiologic factors are another way in which stigma and minority stressors "get under the skin" to affect health. Research on the ways in which minority stressors affect physiologic functioning among LGBT people is still in its relative infancy; however, recent evidence has begun to uncover some of these physiologic mechanisms. Most of this work has focused on alterations in activity of the hypothalamic–pituitary–adrenal (HPA) axis, which is the focus of our review.

Stigma and minority stress may impact regulation of the steroid hormone cortisol, which is released by the HPA axis in response to stressors that are socially threatening.[54] Over time, chronic stress can lead to dysregulation of the HPA axis, which is associated with a host of negative health outcomes, including cardiovascular disease and diabetes.[55] A great deal of work in the general population has established links between social stress, HPA functioning, and health (see[54]), and preliminary evidence suggests that stigma affects HPA axis functioning among sexual minority individuals specifically. For example, researchers recruited 74 LGB young adults who were raised in 24 different states as adolescents. These states differed widely in terms of structural stigma, which was coded based on a composite measure of structural stigma.[38] To examine how prior exposure to structural stigma during adolescence affected subsequent physiologic stress response, participants completed a well-validated laboratory stressor, the Trier Social Stress Test, and neuroendocrine measures were collected. LGB young adults who were raised in high structural stigma states as adolescents evidenced a blunted cortisol response following the Trier Social Stress Test compared with those from low structural stigma states.[56] This pattern of blunted cortisol response has been documented in other groups that have experienced chronic stressors, including children exposed to childhood maltreatment[57] and individuals diagnosed with posttraumatic stress disorder.[58] These results therefore suggest that the stress of growing up in social environments that target gays and lesbians for social exclusion may exert biological effects that are similar to other chronic life stressors.

INTERVENTIONS TO REDUCE STIGMA AND IMPROVE HEALTH AMONG LESBIAN, GAY, BISEXUAL, AND TRANSGENDER YOUTH

Given mounting evidence of the adverse impact of stigma on LGBT health, researchers have begun to develop and test the efficacy of interventions aimed at reducing stigma's health impacts among this population. A recent systematic review identified 43 interventions that either aim to eradicate sexual minority stigma or support sexual minority individuals' abilities to cope with stigma.[59] The majority of these studies were conducted in the past 5 years, suggesting a rapidly increasing momentum to reduce stigma and improve sexual minorities' stigma coping. Just as stigma occurs at different levels of analysis, so too must interventions seek to reduce stigma across these multiple levels. In addition to addressing each of these levels in isolation, it will be important to develop multicomponent interventions, which are likely to be most effective in reducing the negative health consequences of exposure to stigma among LGBT youth.

Structural Interventions

Structural interventions alter the environment so that it contains fewer stressors for LGBT populations. Among youth, this largely takes place within the context of school policies and practices that reduce stigma and prejudice related to sexual orientation and gender identity. A recent study indicated that supportive school climates for LGBT youth may buffer sexual minority youth against risk of suicidality.[60] In this study, information on school climates that protect sexual minority students (eg, percentage of schools with safe spaces and gay–straight alliances, percentage of schools that provided curricula or supplementary materials that included HIV, sexually transmitted diseases, or pregnancy prevention information relevant to LGBT youth) was derived from the School Health Profile Survey, compiled by the Centers for Disease Control and Prevention, and linked to data from the pooled 2005/2007 Youth Risk Behavior Surveillance study from 8 states and cities. LGB students living in the jurisdictions with more protective school climates reported fewer past-year suicidal thoughts than those living in states and cities with less protective climates. Further, sexual orientation disparities in suicidal thoughts were nearly eliminated in states and cities with the most protective school climates.

Another structural-level factor likely to affect the health of LGBT youth is state and district laws and policies that address discrimination, harassment, or bullying of students on the basis of sexual orientation and gender identity.[61] Currently, there are only 19 states with such laws, but promising initial research suggests that comprehensive antibullying policies that specifically include protections for LGBT youth may be effective in reducing risk for suicide attempts among lesbian and gay youth.[62] In this study, researchers coded school district websites and student handbooks across 197 school districts in Oregon to determine whether the districts had any antibullying policies and, if so, whether these policies contained sexual orientation as a protected class status (referred to as "inclusive" policies). These data on antibullying policies were then linked to the Oregon Healthy Teens survey, a population-based dataset of 11th-grade public school students. Lesbian and gay youths living in counties with fewer school districts with inclusive antibullying policies were 2.25 times more likely to have attempted suicide in the past year compared with those living in counties where more districts had these policies.[62]

Finally, structural interventions among LGBT youth are not merely confined to schools. Indeed, broader structural forces that occur outside the school walls—including state laws and policies, but also social attitudes regarding LGBT populations—also powerfully shape the health of LGBT adults and youth,[35] in part because laws and attitudes signal the inherent value of stigmatized groups. Consequently, structural interventions that reduce these broader structural forms of stigma are also needed to improve the health of LGBT youth.

Interpersonal-level and Individual-level Interventions

Interventions at the interpersonal level encourage sexual and gender minority-affirmative interpersonal interactions from parents,[63] mental health providers,[64] and educators.[65] In contrast, individual-level interventions help LGBT individuals to cope with stigma. For example, one of the few stigma coping interventions for sexual minorities to be tested in a randomized controlled trial adapts general cognitive behavioral therapy principles to help young gay and bisexual men identify ongoing sources of stigma-related stress and to rework the negative cognitive, affective, and behavioral tendencies disrupted by this stress.[66] This intervention has yielded significant reductions in depression, alcohol use, and HIV risk behavior among young gay and bisexual men in a waitlist controlled trial[67] and shows strongest effects among those who experience greater levels of minority stress.[68]

FUTURE DIRECTIONS

We highlight 3 key areas for future research. First, research on the stigma–health association, and particularly on mechanisms explaining this association, among transgender youth is lacking relative to research among LGB youth. Given the unique risk and protective factors across these 2 populations, more research is needed to understand whether and how stigma and minority stress may operate differentially among transgender youth compared with LGB youth.

Second, there are several important questions that remain regarding interventions to reduce LGBT health disparities among youth. Despite some progress, most stigma-coping interventions are in early stages of efficacy testing, relying on case studies or pre–post designs without control groups.[69–71] Stronger tests of these interventions are needed to establish stronger causal inferences. Further, structural interventions (eg, changing laws and policies) cannot typically be tested in randomized controlled trials for ethical reasons; thus, the field requires more prospective, quasiexperimental designs to test these interventions. Additionally, the Internet and social media are increasingly being used for the delivery of health interventions, including among LGBT populations.[72] The application of these technologies to LGBT health interventions among youth requires further investigation.

Third, prejudice among health care providers, as well as structural aspects of the medical institution itself, may compromise the quality of care that LGBT youth receive. Indeed, many medical providers lack confidence in their knowledge of sexual minority health,[73] with nearly one-half of all medical students reporting unease about treating sexual minority clients.[74] One reason for such discomfort is that medical students receive an average of only 2.5 to 5 hours of training about sexual minority health,[75] with one-third of medical schools providing 0 hours of clinical training related to sexual minority health.[74] Medical providers and students report being even more unprepared and uncomfortable in discussing transgender health issues, including sex reassignment surgery and gender transitioning,[76] with nearly one-half of transgender individuals in 1 national study reporting that they had to teach their provider about transgender care.[77] Few studies, however, have examined the impact of stigma reduction efforts specifically in health care settings, such as the development of policies barring sexual orientation and gender identity discrimination in hospitals on patient outcomes, and of evidence-based practices so that all medical care staff (eg, receptionists, medical assistants, clinicians) can deliver affirming communications and appropriate care with LGBT youth. Examining the influence of provider attitudes, both implicit and explicit, on health outcomes among LGBT youth represents another important research avenue.

SUMMARY

Stigma occurs at multiple levels—including individual (eg, concealment), interpersonal (eg, victimization), and structural (eg, laws and policies)—to affect the health of LGBT youth. Stigma at each of these levels disrupts several cognitive (eg, vigilance), affective (eg, rumination), interpersonal (eg, social isolation), and physiologic (eg, stress reactivity) processes that in turn influence health. Several of these stigma-inducing mechanisms can be targeted in both clinical and public health interventions to reduce LGBT health disparities among youth, and emerging evidence suggests the efficacy of such interventions, although more research is needed.

At first glance, it may seem that the topic of stigma and minority stress falls outside the purview of the medical profession. After all, medical doctors are trained to deal with disease-specific processes rather than interpersonal and structural factors that affect their patients. However, as noted, the medical profession has generated stigma against LGBT youth at both the interpersonal and structural levels,[1] and therefore has an important role to play in improving the health of this population. Awareness of stigma and minority stress as etiologic factors contributing to the disproportionate burden of adverse mental and physical health outcomes among LGBT youth is essential to the provision of appropriate care for this population, such as making referrals to mental health providers when warranted. Moreover, pediatricians can become effective advocates for LGBT youth and their families in addressing barriers to poor health that occur outside the confines of the medical office. Finally, to the extent that the health care profession itself is a source of stigma for LGBT youth, pediatricians can take a leading role in efforts to develop and evaluate stigma-reduction efforts within the health care setting to improve the health of LGBT youth.

REFERENCES

1. Institute of Medicine. The health of lesbian, gay, bisexual, and transgender people: building a foundation for better understanding. Washington, DC: The National Academies Press; 2011.
2. Link BG, Phelan JC. Conceptualizing stigma. Annu Rev Sociol 2001;27:363–85.

3. Meyer IH. Prejudice, social stress, and mental health in lesbian, gay, and bisexual populations: conceptual issues and research evidence. Psychol Bull 2003; 129(5):674–97.
4. Lick DJ, Durso LE, Johnson KL. Minority stress and physical health among sexual minorities. Perspect Psychol Sci 2013;8(5):521–48.
5. Operario D, Yang MF, Reisner SL, et al. Stigma and the syndemic of HIV-related health risk behaviors in a diverse sample of transgender women. J Community Psychol 2014;42(5):544–57.
6. White-Hughto JM, Reisner SL, Pachankis JE. Stigma and transgender health: a critical review of stigma determinants, mechanisms, and interventions in U.S. transgender populations. Soc Sci Med 2015;147:222–31.
7. Weber G. Using to numb the pain: substance use and abuse among lesbian, gay, and bisexual individuals. J Ment Health Couns 2008;30(1):31–48.
8. Hatzenbuehler ML, Nolen-Hoeksema S, Erickson SJ. Minority stress predictors of HIV risk behavior, substance use, and depressive symptoms: results from a prospective study of bereaved gay men. Health Psychol 2008;27(4):455–62.
9. Reilly A, Rudd NA. Is internalized homonegativity related to body image? Fam Consum Sci Res J 2006;35(1):58–73.
10. Rosario M, Schrimshaw EW, Hunter J. A model of sexual risk behaviors among young gay and bisexual men: longitudinal associations of mental health, substance abuse, sexual abuse, and the coming-out process. AIDS Educ Prev 2006;18(5):444.
11. Perez-Brumer A, Hatzenbuehler ML, Oldenburg CE, et al. Individual-and structural-level risk factors for suicide attempts among transgender adults. Behav Med 2015;41(3):164–71.
12. Mendoza-Denton R, Downey G, Purdie VJ, et al. Sensitivity to status-based rejection: implications for African American students' college experience. J Pers Soc Psychol 2002;83(4):896.
13. Westenberg PM, Drewes MJ, Goedhart AW, et al. A developmental analysis of self-reported fears in late childhood through mid- adolescence: social-evaluative fears on the rise? J Child Psychol Psychiatry 2004;45(3):481–95.
14. Lev-Wiesel R, Nuttman-Shwartz O, Sternberg R. Peer rejection during adolescence: psychological long-term effects—a brief report. J Loss Trauma 2006; 11(2):131–42.
15. Downey G, Bonica C, Rincon C. Rejection sensitivity and adolescent romantic relationships. The Development Romantic Relationships Adolescence. Cambridge, UK: Cambridge University Press; 1999. p. 148–74.
16. Cole SW, Kemeny ME, Taylor SE. Social identity and physical health: accelerated HIV progression in rejection-sensitive gay men. J Pers Soc Psychol 1997;72(2):320.
17. Wang K, Rendina HJ, Pachankis JE. Gay-related rejection sensitivity as a risk factor for condomless sex. AIDS Behav 2016;20(4):763–7.
18. Pachankis JE. The psychological implications of concealing a stigma: a cognitive-affective-behavioral model. Psychol Bull 2007;133(2):328.
19. Pachankis JE, Cochran SD, Mays VM. The mental health of sexual minority adults in and out of the closet: a population-based study. J Consult Clin Psychol 2015; 83(5):890.
20. Frost DM, Bastone LM. The role of stigma concealment in the retrospective high school experiences of gay, lesbian, and bisexual individuals. J LGBT Youth 2008; 5(1):27–36.
21. Frable DE, Platt L, Hoey S. Concealable stigmas and positive self-perceptions: feeling better around similar others. J Pers Soc Psychol 1998;74(4):909.

22. Frable DE, Wortman C, Joseph J. Predicting self-esteem, well-being, and distress in a cohort of gay men: the importance of cultural stigma, personal visibility, community networks, and positive identity. J Pers 1997;65(3):599–624.
23. Ragins BR, Singh R, Cornwell JM. Making the invisible visible: fear and disclosure of sexual orientation at work. J Appl Psychol 2007;92(4):1103.
24. Petroll AE, Mosack KE. Physician awareness of sexual orientation and preventive health recommendations to men who have sex with men. Sex Transm Dis 2011; 38(1):63.
25. Cochran SD. Emerging issues in research on lesbians' and gay men's mental health: does sexual orientation really matter? Am Psychol 2001;56(11):931.
26. Cohen-Kettenis PT, van Goozen SH. Adolescents who are eligible for sex reassignment surgery: parental reports of emotional and behavioural problems. Clin Child Psychol Psychiatry 2002;7(3):412–22.
27. Reisner SL, White-Hughto JM, Dunham EE, et al. Legal protections in public accommodations settings: a critical public health issue for transgender and gender-nonconforming people. Milbank Q 2015;93(3):484–515.
28. Gagné P, Tewksbury R. Conformity pressures and gender resistance among transgendered individuals. Soc Probl 1998;45:81–101.
29. Samuel L, Zaritsky E. Communicating effectively with transgender patients. Am Fam Physician 2008;78(5):648–50.
30. Alegria CA. Transgender identity and health care: implications for psychosocial and physical evaluation. J Am Acad Nurse Pract 2011;23(4):175–82.
31. Herek GM. Hate crimes and stigma-related experiences among sexual minority adults in the United States: prevalence estimates from a national probability sample. J Interpers Violence 2009;24(1):54–74.
32. Woodford MR, Howell ML, Kulick A, et al. "That's so gay" heterosexual male undergraduates and the perpetuation of sexual orientation microaggressions on campus. J Interpers Violence 2013;28(2):416–35.
33. Hatzenbuehler ML, Link BG. Introduction to the special issue on structural stigma and health. Soc Sci Med 2014;103:1–6.
34. Hatzenbuehler ML. Structural stigma and the health of lesbian, gay, and bisexual populations. Curr Dir Psychol Sci 2014;23(2):127–32.
35. Duncan DT, Hatzenbuehler ML. Lesbian, gay, bisexual, and transgender hate crimes and suicidality among a population-based sample of sexual-minority adolescents in Boston. Am J Public Health 2014;104(2):272–8.
36. Hatzenbuehler ML, Duncan DT, Johnson RM. Neighborhood-level LGBT hate crimes and bullying among sexual minority youths: a geospatial analysis. Violence Vict 2015;30(4):663–75.
37. Duncan DT, Hatzenbuehler ML, Johnson RM. Neighborhood-level LGBT hate crimes and current illicit drug use among sexual minority youth. Drug Alcohol Depend 2014;135:65–70.
38. Hatzenbuehler ML. The social environment and suicide attempts in lesbian, gay, and bisexual youth. Pediatrics 2011;127(5):896–903.
39. Hatzenbuehler ML, Jun H-J, Corliss HL, et al. Structural stigma and cigarette smoking in a prospective cohort study of sexual minority and heterosexual youth. Ann Behav Med 2014;47(1):48–56.
40. Hatzenbuehler ML, Jun H-J, Corliss HL, et al. Structural stigma and sexual orientation disparities in adolescent drug use. Addict Behav 2015;46:14–8.
41. Hatzenbuehler ML. How does sexual minority stigma "get under the skin"? a psychological mediation framework. Psychol Bull 2009;135(5):707.

42. Hatzenbuehler ML, Phelan JC, Link BG. Stigma as a fundamental cause of population health inequalities. Am J Public Health 2013;103(5):813–21.
43. Crocker J, Major B, Steele C. Social stigma. In: Gilbert D, Fiske S, Lindzey G, editors. The handbook of social psychology, Vol. 2. Boston, MA: McGraw-Hill; 1998. p. 504–53.
44. Gump BB, Matthews KA. Vigilance and cardiovascular reactivity to subsequent stressors in men: a preliminary study. Health Psychol 1998;17(1):93.
45. Pachankis JE, Goldfried MR, Ramrattan ME. Extension of the rejection sensitivity construct to the interpersonal functioning of gay men. J Consult Clin Psychol 2008;76(2):306.
46. Gross JJ. Emotion regulation in adulthood: timing is everything. Curr Dir Psychol Sci 2001;10(6):214–9.
47. Nolen-Hoeksema S. Responses to depression and their effects on the duration of depressive episodes. J Abnorm Psychol 1991;100(4):569.
48. McLaughlin KA, Hatzenbuehler ML, Hilt LM. Emotion dysregulation as a mechanism linking peer victimization to internalizing symptoms in adolescents. J Consult Clin Psychol 2009;77(5):894.
49. Hatzenbuehler ML, McLaughlin KA, Nolen-Hoeksema S. Emotion regulation and internalizing symptoms in a longitudinal study of sexual minority and heterosexual adolescents. J Child Psychol Psychiatry 2008;49(12):1270–8.
50. Hatzenbuehler ML, Nolen-Hoeksema S, Dovidio J. How does stigma "get under the skin"? The mediating role of emotion regulation. Psychol Sci 2009;20(10): 1282–9.
51. Cacioppo S, Grippo AJ, London S, et al. Loneliness clinical import and interventions. Perspect Psychol Sci 2015;10(2):238–49.
52. Ryan C, Russell ST, Huebner D, et al. Family acceptance in adolescence and the health of LGBT young adults. J Child Adolesc Psychiatr Nurs 2010;23(4):205–13.
53. Kelly AE. Clients' secret keeping in outpatient therapy. J Couns Psychol 1998; 45(1):50.
54. Dickerson SS, Kemeny ME. Acute stressors and cortisol responses: a theoretical integration and synthesis of laboratory research. Psychol Bull 2004;130(3):355.
55. Lundberg U. Stress hormones in health and illness: the roles of work and gender. Psychoneuroendocrinology 2005;30(10):1017–21.
56. Hatzenbuehler ML, McLaughlin KA. Structural stigma and hypothalamic–pituitary–adrenocortical axis reactivity in lesbian, gay, and bisexual young adults. Ann Behav Med 2014;47(1):39–47.
57. Gunnar MR, Frenn K, Wewerka SS, et al. Moderate versus severe early life stress: associations with stress reactivity and regulation in 10-12 year-old children. Psychoneuroendocrinology 2009;34(1):62–75.
58. Yehuda R, Bierer LM, Schmeidler J, et al. Low cortisol and risk for PTSD in adult offspring of holocaust survivors. Am J Psychiatry 2000;157(8):1252–9.
59. Chaudoir S, Wang K, Pachankis JE. What reduces sexual minority stress? A review of the intervention toolkit. Unpublished Manuscript, College of the Holy Cross, Worcester, MA; 2016.
60. Hatzenbuehler ML, Birkett M, Van Wagenen A, et al. Protective school climates and reduced risk for suicide ideation in sexual minority youths. Am J Public Health 2014;104(2):279–86.
61. Movement Advancement Project. Safe Schools Laws. 2015. Available at: http://www.lgbtmap.org/equality-maps/safe_school_laws. Accessed June 7, 2015.
62. Hatzenbuehler ML, Keyes KM. Inclusive anti-bullying policies and reduced risk of suicide attempts in lesbian and gay youth. J Adolesc Health 2013;53(1):S21–6.

63. Huebner DM, Rullo JE, Thoma BC, et al. Piloting lead with love: a film-based intervention to improve parents' responses to their lesbian, gay, and bisexual children. J Prim Prev 2013;34(5):359–69.
64. Rutter PA, Estrada D, Ferguson LK, et al. Sexual orientation and counselor competency: the impact of training on enhancing awareness, knowledge and skills. J LGBT Issues Couns 2008;2(2):109–25.
65. Greytak EA, Kosciw JG, Boesen MJ. Educating the educator: creating supportive school personnel through professional development. J Sch Violence 2013;12(1): 80–97.
66. Pachankis JE. Uncovering clinical principles and techniques to address minority stress, mental health, and related health risks among gay and bisexual men. Clin Psychol (New York) 2014;21(4):313–30.
67. Pachankis JE, Hatzenbuehler ML, Rendina HJ, et al. LGB-Affirmative cognitive-behavioral therapy for young adult gay and bisexual men: a randomized controlled trial of a transdiagnostic minority stress approach. J Consult Clin Psychol 2015;83(5):875–89.
68. Millar B, Wang K, Pachankis JE. The moderating role of implicit internalized homonegativity on the efficacy of LGB-affirmative psychotherapy: results from a randomized controlled trial with young adult gay and bisexual men. J Consult Clin Psychol 2016;84(7):565–70.
69. Craig SL, Austin A, Alessi E. Gay affirmative cognitive behavioral therapy for sexual minority youth: a clinical adaptation. Clin Soc Work J 2013;41(3):258–66.
70. Diamond GM, Diamond GS, Levy S, et al. Attachment-based family therapy for suicidal lesbian, gay, and bisexual adolescents: a treatment development study and open trial with preliminary findings. Psychotherapy 2012;49(1):62–71.
71. LaSala M. Cognitive and environmental intervention for gay males: addressing stigma and its consequences. Fam Soc 2006;87(2):181–9.
72. Mustanski B, Greene GJ, Ryan D, et al. Feasibility, acceptability, and initial efficacy of an online sexual health promotion program for LGBT youth: the queer sex Ed intervention. J Sex Res 2015;52(2):220–30.
73. Anderson S, McNair R, Mitchell A. Addressing health inequalities in Victorian lesbian, gay, bisexual and transgender communities. Health Promot J Austr 2001;11(1):32–8.
74. Obedin-Maliver J, Goldsmith ES, Stewart L, et al. Lesbian, gay, bisexual, and transgender–related content in undergraduate medical education. JAMA 2011; 306(9):971–7.
75. McGarry KA, Clarke JG, Cyr MG, et al. Evaluating a lesbian and gay health care curriculum. Teach Learn Med 2002;14(4):244–8.
76. White W, Brenman S, Paradis E, et al. Lesbian, Gay, Bisexual, and Transgender Patient Care: Medical Students' Preparedness and Comfort. Teach Learn Med 2015;27(3):254–63.
77. Grant M, Mottet L, Tanis J, et al. National transgender discrimination survey report on health and health care. Washington, DC: National Center for Transgender Equality and National Gay and Lesbian Task Force; 2010.

Bullying Among Lesbian, Gay, Bisexual, and Transgender Youth

 CrossMark

Valerie A. Earnshaw, PhD[a,b,*], Laura M. Bogart, PhD[a,b,c],
V. Paul Poteat, PhD[d], Sari L. Reisner, ScD[a,b,e,f],
Mark A. Schuster, MD, PhD[a,b]

KEYWORDS

- Bullying • Gender expression • Gender identity • Healthcare • LGBT
- Peer victimization • Sexual orientation • Youth

KEY POINTS

- Bullying of lesbian, gay, bisexual, and transgender (LGBT) youth is prevalent in the United States; the majority of LGBT youth experience some form of bullying.
- Bullying undermines the mental, behavioral, and physical health of LGBT youth, with consequences lasting into adulthood.
- Pediatricians can play a vital role in promoting the well-being of LGBT youth by preventing and identifying bullying, offering counsel to youth and their parents, and advocating for programs and policies.

INTRODUCTION

Bullying of lesbian, gay, bisexual, and transgender (LGBT) youth persists in the United States, with harmful and sometimes fatal consequences. Media reports about LGBT youth who have died by suicide frequently describe experiences of bullying victimization. For example, after being the target of bullying for several years, Adam Kizer died

Disclosure Statement: Dr V.A. Earnshaw's effort was supported by the Agency for Healthcare Research and Quality (AHRQ; K12 HS022986). Drs L.M. Bogart, V.P. Poteat, S.L. Reisner, and M.A. Schuster have nothing to disclose.
[a] Division of General Pediatrics, Boston Children's Hospital, 300 Longwood Ave, Boston, MA 02115, USA; [b] Department of Pediatrics, Harvard Medical School, 300 Longwood Ave, Boston, MA 02115, USA; [c] Health Unit, RAND Corporation, 1776 Main Street, P.O. Box 2138 Santa Monica, CA 90407-2138, USA; [d] Counseling, Developmental, and Educational Psychology Department, Boston College, 140 Commonwealth Ave, Campion Hall 307, Chestnut Hill, MA 02467, USA; [e] Department of Epidemiology, Harvard T.H. Chan School of Public Health, 677 Huntington Ave, Boston, MA 02115, USA; [f] The Fenway Institute, Fenway Health, 1340 Boylston Street, Boston, MA 02215, USA
* Corresponding author. Boston Children's Hospital, 21 Autumn Street, Room 212.1, Boston, MA 02115.
E-mail address: valerie.earnshaw@childrens.harvard.edu

by suicide at age 16, 6 months after coming out as bisexual. Adam's father reported that he was bullied starting at age 9, when his peers identified him as "different."[1] Adam suffered substantial mistreatment from his peers that was both verbal (eg, suggestions that he should kill himself) and physical (eg, tied to a tree, doused in gasoline, and almost set on fire). Another example is that of Taylor Alesana, a young transgender woman who experienced significant bullying victimization at school and online, and died by suicide at age 16.[2,3] She described social isolation and rejection on Transgender Day of Remembrance, stating in a YouTube video: "Finding friends when you're transgender, that to me is one of the hardest parts because you don't find a lot of friends. And when you do, a lot of them will leave you just because you're different."[3] The ridiculing comments on YouTube continued even after Taylor's suicide.[4]

Adam and Taylor's experiences of bullying by peers are common among LGBT youth. Although extreme in their consequences, these examples underscore the need to address bullying of LGBT youth. Pediatricians can play an important role in preventing and reporting LGBT bullying, supporting LGBT youth who are bullied, and promoting the health and well-being of LGBT youth. In this article, we define key concepts relevant to LGBT bullying; discuss its prevalence in the United States; review evidence of its psychological, behavioral, and physical health consequences; and make recommendations for how pediatricians can address it.

KEY CONCEPTS

Sexual orientation is a relational construct involving a pattern of romantic relationships with, or desires for, people of a particular gender.[5] Sexual orientation is inclusive of *behavior* (eg, whether individuals are sexually engaged with same-gender and/or opposite-gender partners), *identity* (eg, how individuals understand and represent themselves based on identities such as "gay," "lesbian," "bisexual," or "heterosexual"), and/or *attraction* or desire.[6] The first 3 letters of the LGBT abbreviation (LGB; lesbian, gay, bisexual) refer to a range of sexual minority orientations that are not exclusively heterosexual. We include individuals who are "queer" or "questioning" under the LGBT umbrella.

Gender identity is one's internal sense of being male, female, or outside these categories, and gender expression is the manifestation of culturally defined feminine or masculine traits in personality, appearance, and behavior.[5,7] The last letter of the LGBT abbreviation (T; transgender) refers to a range of gender minority identities and expressions that are not aligned exclusively with one's assigned sex at birth. Some LGBT people display a nonconforming gender expression during development; some do not. Children with a conforming gender expression may grow up to be LGB or heterosexual; they may be transgender or they may not. People have a sexual orientation, gender identity, and gender expression, and these are related in complex ways throughout youth development (for a discussion of the development of sexual orientation and gender, including their associations, see Stewart L. Adelson and colleagues' article, "Development and Mental Health of LGBT Youth in Pediatric Practice," in this issue).

Having perceived to have a minority sexual orientation, gender identity, and/or gender expression may increase youths' risk of being bullying. *Bullying* is defined by the Centers for Disease Control and Prevention and US Department of Education as:

> *Bullying is any unwanted aggressive behavior(s) by another youth or group of youths who are not siblings or current dating partners that involves an observed or perceived power imbalance and is repeated multiple times or is highly likely to be repeated. Bullying may inflict harm or distress on the targeted youth including physical, psychological, or educational harm.[8]*

This definition emphasizes that bullying behavior is unwanted, meaning that the bullied youth wants the behavior to stop. It is aggressive, meaning that it involves the intentional use of harmful behavior. A power imbalance refers to a real or perceived ability of the perpetrator to control the target's behaviors or outcomes. Power can be drawn from a variety of sources, such as physical strength, popularity, or wealth. Incidents are considered repeated if they occur multiple times or there is a concern that they are likely to recur. Moreover, bullying may result in harm involving negative experiences or injuries.

Mistreatment of LGBT youth is also referred to by other terms in the literature, including discrimination and bias. Although we use the term bullying in this article, we acknowledge that LGBT bullying is stigma-based and therefore fundamentally discriminatory in nature.

SCOPE OF PROBLEM

Data from US national samples suggest that the majority of LGBT youth experience some form of bullying. In 2011, the Gay, Lesbian and Straight Education Network surveyed more than 8500 LGBT youth aged 13–20 years old in all 50 US states and Washington DC.[9] All forms of bullying were prevalent among these youth (**Table 1**). Most (92.3%) reported experiencing *verbal bullying*, involving harmful oral or written communication including taunting, name calling, and threats. Close to one-half (44.7%) reported *physical bullying*, including the use of physical force such as hitting, kicking, tripping, and spitting. About one-fifth (21.2%) reported more extreme physical assault, such as being punched, kicked, or injured with a weapon. Most (89.5%) reported *social or relational bullying*, involving behavior intended to harm reputations and relationships including spreading rumors, posting embarrassing media content, and socially isolating the target. Nearly one-half (47.7%) reported *damage to property*, such as stealing, damaging, or altering property. More than one-half of youth (55.2%) reported bullying via technology, or *cyberbullying*. Although youth attributed experiences of bullying to multiple socially devalued characteristics (eg, religion,

Table 1
Types of bullying and prevalence among LGBT youth in the United States

Type	Definition	Examples	Prevalence Among LGBT Youth in Past Year (%)[a]
Verbal	Harmful oral or written communication	Taunting, name calling, threatening	92.3
Physical	Use of physical force	Hitting, kicking, tripping, spitting	44.7
Social or relational	Behavior intended to harm reputations or relationships	Spreading rumors, posting embarrassing media content, isolating socially	89.5
Damage to property	Stealing, damaging, or altering property	Stealing or deleting electronic information	47.7

Abbreviation: LGBT, lesbian, gay, bisexual, and transgender.
[a] Estimates of prevalence are from the US national 2011 National School Climate Survey conducted by the Gay, Lesbian, & Straight Education Network.[9]

race/ethnicity, disability), they attributed the majority of bullying to their sexual orientation or gender expression. Other data sources suggest similarly high prevalence estimates of bullying among LGBT youth.[10]

LGBT youth generally experience more bullying than non-LGBT youth. In an online study of youth ages 13 to 18 years, LGB youth reported more than twice as much online and in-person peer victimization as heterosexual youth.[11] Moreover, these different rates of bullying seem to begin before youth generally identify as LGB: youth who identify as LGB in 10th grade are more likely to have reported bullying than non-LGB youth when they were in 5th grade.[12] Similar differences are documented for transgender youth: approximately 83% of transgender or gender nonconforming youth reported bullying victimization in the past year in comparison with 58% of cisgender (ie, nontransgender) youth in a recent study.[13] Adolescent boys who are bullied because they are perceived to be gay owing to nonconforming gender expression (even if they do not identify as gay themselves) also experience more verbal and physical bullying than boys who are bullied for other reasons.[14]

Although understudied, some work suggests variability in the prevalence of bullying among LGBT youth. For example, LGBT youth who have disclosed their sexual orientation or gender identity to their peers or school staff report greater bullying relative to youth who have not disclosed their LGBT status,[9,15] although it is possible that LGBT youth who are bullied are more likely to disclose to adults and be discovered as being LGBT by peers. Youth who identify as bisexual also seem to report greater bullying.[16] The prevalence of bullying also seems to vary by social context. LGBT youth report more bullying in states that do not have laws that prohibit bullying or harassment on the basis of sexual orientation or gender identity, and LGBT youth in the Midwest and South report more bullying than youth in the North and West.[9] Moreover, LGB youth who live in neighborhoods with high rates of LGBT assault hate crimes are more likely to report relational and cyberbullying, possibly because violence toward LGBT adults in neighborhoods signals acceptance of LGBT bullying.[17]

CAUSES AND CONSEQUENCES OF LESBIAN, GAY, BISEXUAL, AND TRANSGENDER BULLYING

Multiple factors contribute to youths' engagement in bullying against LGBT individuals. At the societal level, LGBT stigma (social devaluation and discrediting of LGBT people) leads to discrimination and bullying of LGBT youth (see Mark L. Hatzenbuehler and John E. Pachankis' article, "Stigma and Minority Stress as Social Determinants of Health among LGBT Youth: Research Evidence and Clinical Implications," in this issue). At the social level, youth socialize and influence LGBT bullying within their peer groups. Certain norms within peer groups contribute to greater LGBT bullying, including traditional masculinity norms, dominance norms, and overall aggression levels.[18,19] Having fewer LGBT friends is associated with greater engagement in LGBT bullying. At the individual level, a prominent contributing factor is prejudice, or negative attitudes toward others based on their minority sexual orientation and/or gender identity and expression that are rooted in LGBT stigma.[20,21] Greater engagement in LGBT bullying is also associated with holding stronger attitudes in support of social dominance, hierarchies, and power differentials among peers as well as at a broader societal level against socially devalued groups (eg, racial minorities, women).[22] Heterosexual youth who place greater importance on their heterosexual identity as part of their overall sense of identity and those who are less empathic tend to perpetrate more LGBT bullying.[20] Boys tend to engage in LGBT bullying more than girls. Also, youth who engage in bullying in general are more likely to perpetrate LGBT bullying specifically.[20]

LGBT bullying undermines the mental, behavioral, and physical health of youth, ultimately leading to health inequities for LGBT compared with non-LGBT youth that may last across the lifespan. As highlighted in the introduction, suicidal ideation and suicide attempts and completion are a concern for youth experiencing LGBT bullying. Sexual minority youth are more likely to think about and attempt suicide than non-LGBT youth, and bullying plays a role in these thoughts and behaviors.[23,24] Other mental health effects of LGBT bullying include greater symptoms of depression and anxiety, and lower self-esteem.[9,23,24] Longitudinal evidence among youth in general suggests that bullying is associated with worse mental health outcomes over time, with past experiences of bullying predicting worse psychosocial quality of life, more depression symptoms, and worse self-worth.[25] Some evidence suggests that youth who disclose their sexual orientation or gender identity to school peers and staff report greater psychological well-being than those youth who do not, despite experiencing greater bullying.[9] It is possible that youth who choose to disclose a sexual or gender minority status at school gain resilience resources, such as social support, after disclosing. More research is needed to understand associations among disclosure, bullying, and well-being, including the ways in which resilience resources and supportive environments affect these associations.

Bullying plays a role in harmful health behaviors among LGBT youth. LGBT bullying is associated with greater engagement in substance use, including tobacco, alcohol, marijuana, and other illicit drugs (eg, methamphetamines, inhalants).[13,26] It is also associated with engagement in risk behaviors related to substance use, such as drunk driving.[26] Although the topic is understudied, LGBT youth who are bullied may engage in high levels of sexual risk behaviors (eg, condomless sex, substance use before sex, transactional sex), similar to LGBT adults.[27,28] Also of concern, LGBT middle and high school students who experience greater bullying have higher rates of school absenteeism (often related to fears of being bullied at school), lower grade point averages, and lower postgraduation educational aspirations.[9]

Bullying further affects the physical health of LGBT youth. LGBT youth who are physically bullied may suffer cuts, bruises, broken bones, and other direct health sequelae of physical violence. Other physical health outcomes are understudied among LGBT youth specifically, but a robust body of research describes outcomes of bullying among youth in general. Youth who experience bullying are more likely to experience a range of physical health symptoms, including increased abdominal pain, headache, poor appetite, sleeping problems, and skin problems, as well as greater body mass index, higher systolic and diastolic blood pressures, and decreased self-rated health, relative to youth who are not bullied.[29,30,31,32] These health outcomes seem to be driven, in part, by the mental and behavioral health consequences of bullying.[30] That is, similar to the ways in which discrimination affects health among adults,[33] depression, anxiety, and other poor mental health effects of bullying may lead to worse physical health. Additionally, youth may engage in harmful coping behaviors (eg, substance use to manage anxiety), which ultimately undermine physical health.

The consequences of bullying among LGBT youth seem to be worse than the consequences among non-LGBT youth. Youth who experience LGBT-based bullying engage in greater substance use and other risk behaviors (eg, drunk driving), and experience higher rates of depression than youth who experience bullying that is not bias-based.[26] Similarly, adolescent boys who are bullied because they are perceived to be gay experience greater anxiety and depressive symptoms than boys bullied for other reasons.[14]

Although rates of bullying among LGBT youth seem to decrease with age,[12,34] the mental, behavioral, and physical health consequences of bullying may last into adulthood. LGBT young adults who self-report frequent bullying as adolescents are more likely to be depressed, have had a suicide attempt, engage in sexual risk behaviors including condomless sex, and be diagnosed with a sexually transmitted infection.[15,34,35] Similarly, adults who experienced bullying associated with having a nonconforming gender expression as youth report greater depressive symptoms and lower life satisfaction as young adults.[36,37] LGBT adults who experienced greater bullying as youth are more likely to report posttraumatic stress disorder.[38]

RECOMMENDATIONS FOR CLINICIANS

Pediatricians and other clinicians practicing pediatric care have an opportunity and professional responsibility to address LGBT bullying to improve the well-being of LGBT youth. Here, we make recommendations to pediatricians regarding how to address LGBT bullying with patients and parents as well as within communities. We focus on LGBT bullying, but many of these recommendations generalize to other forms of bullying. These recommendations are largely guided by the American Academy of Pediatrics,[39] American Medical Association,[40] and the US Department of Health and Human Services.[41,42] It may also be useful for pediatricians to learn about local policies on bullying to help individual youth and their families navigate bullying at school. Pediatricians may contact representatives of school districts (eg, principals, guidance counselors, school nurses) and explore school websites for more information on school bullying policies. Some states also have laws that protect students from bullying on the basis of sexual orientation and gender identity. The Gay, Lesbian and Straight Education Network maintains state-specific resource guides on local bullying policies that may be useful for pediatricians.[43] In addition, Title IX has been used in several legal cases related to students experiencing discrimination on the basis of gender expression.[44]

Several of our recommendations encourage pediatricians to work with other adults, including parents, teachers, school administrators, and other community stakeholders, to address LGBT bullying. It is important for pediatricians to bear in mind that these other adults may actively or passively mistreat LGBT youth (eg, use antigay epithets to mock gay students, ignore bullying).[45] Societal LGBT stigma leads both youth and adults to discriminate against LGBT youth. Pediatricians must be sensitive to this issue. In some cases, it may be possible for pediatricians to identify and work with other accepting adults to support LGBT youth. In other cases, when accepting adults are not present within youths' lives, it is critical for pediatricians to act as allies of and advocates for LGBT youth experiencing bullying to promote their well-being (eg, by connecting them to community-based health or social organizations that are LGBT affirming).

Box 1 suggests several steps that pediatricians can take to address bullying. Importantly, addressing bullying starts with *prevention*. Pediatricians can include bullying in anticipatory guidance by describing bullying and its consequences to parents and youth.[45] They can describe what bullying is, and what forms it may take. Pediatricians can also discuss techniques to address bullying with youth (eg, tell an adult) so that youth are prepared to respond to bullying should they witness or experience it. Pediatricians can also encourage parents to promote positive social skills among youth (eg, nonaggressive behavior).[46] Any youth may experience LGBT-related bullying—not only those who are LGBT—based on perceived sexual orientation or gender identity. Pediatricians therefore should not limit their discussion of LGBT bullying to youth who are LGBT themselves. Similarly, LGBT youth may experience many forms of

---

Box 1
Steps for pediatricians to address LGBT bullying

Prevent

- Describe bullying and its consequences to parents and youth.
- Discuss ways to safely respond to bullying.

Identify

- Create safe environment in which youth feel comfortable discussing sexual orientation and gender identity.
- Screen youth for bullying.
- Identify type of bullying and youth involved.

Counsel

- Help youth to identify accepting and supportive adults.
- Advise parents on how to advocate for youth in school.

Advocate

- Speak out against LGBT bullying and stigma.
- Advocate for policies to address LGBT bullying and stigma.

Abbreviation: LGBT, lesbian, gay, bisexual, and transgender.

---

bullying, such as based on race or disability. Pediatricians should not limit their discussions with LGBT youth to LGBT bullying, but instead discuss all forms of bullying.

Pediatricians should seek to *identify* youth who are targets of LGBT bullying. This is particularly important because many LGBT youth do not disclose their experiences of bullying to other adults, including teachers.[9] LGBT youth report not telling teachers about bullying because they are concerned about teachers' reactions, they fear making the situation worse, and they feel that teachers will not effectively address the situation.[9]

Pediatricians can contribute to the creation of safe and welcoming spaces wherein LGBT youth feel comfortable discussing LGBT bullying (see Scott E. Hadland and colleagues' article, "Caring for LGBTQ Youth in Inclusive and Affirmative Environments," in this issue). Although LGB youth often do not disclose their sexual orientation to their physicians, many report that they would be open to discussing it if the subject were raised by their physician.[47] When seeking to identify bullying, pediatricians should pay particular attention to LGBT youth, who are at increased risk of experiencing bullying, and youth exhibiting mental, behavioral, or physical symptoms of bullying (eg, anxiety, substance use, unexplained physical injury).[45] Physicians may ask both youth and parents about bullying. Example questions to identify bullying are included in **Box 2**. Direct questions ask about bullying explicitly, whereas indirect questions are meant to generate conversation that may provide insight into bullying. If patients or parents indicate that patients have experienced bullying, pediatricians may ask follow-up questions to gain more information and determine whether it is LGBT bullying. For example, they should listen to see whether homophobic epithets are involved in the bullying or whether the youth attributes bullying to their real or perceived sexual minority orientation, gender nonconforming behavior, or transgender identity.

Pediatricians should provide counsel to youth who are experiencing LGBT bullying. Pediatricians can advise youth regarding how to react if they are bullied, including by

---

Box 2
Suggested questions for pediatricians to ask youth and caregivers to identify youth who might be experiencing bullying

Youth

Direct
- Have you been bullied by other kids?
- Have you been teased or left out by other kids?
- Have other kids spread rumors about you?
- Have you been hurt, punched, or kicked by other kids?
- Have other kids taken or damaged anything that belongs to you?

Indirect
- What is lunch time like at your school? Whom do you sit with?
- What is it like to ride the school bus?

Follow-up
- Could you describe a time when you were bullied?
- What did the other kids say?
- What did the other kids do?
- Why do you think that they are treating you this way?

Caregivers

Direct
- Do you suspect that your child is being bullied or harassed?
- Is your child bothered by other kids?
- Does your child have problems with other kids?

Indirect
- How does your child get along with other kids?
- Does your child have many friends?
- Is your child nervous about going to school?

Adapted from Get Help Now. Stopbullying.gov Web site. Available at: http://www.stopbullying.gov/get-help-now/index.html. Accessed October 26, 2015; and Glew G, Rivara F, Feudtner C. Bullying: children hurting children. Pediatrics Rev 2000;21(6):183–9.

---

staying calm, walking away, and telling an adult.[41] Pediatricians can help youth to identify supportive adults (eg, parents, teachers, school administrators) to whom they can turn when bullied. Teachers involved in gay–straight alliances, for example, may be advocates for LGBT students. LGBT youth report that social support received from these adults at school helps them cope with bullying.[48] In addition, pediatricians can provide support for youth who decide to tell their parents or other adults about experiences of LGBT bullying. Pediatricians can further encourage youth to join safe and supportive extracurricular activities to reduce social isolation and strengthen their relationships with others.

Pediatricians can also counsel parents of youth who are experiencing LGBT bullying. If the pediatrician has learned of the bullying through a private, confidential conversation with the youth, he or she cannot tell parents about a patients' experiences of bullying without permission unless the patient is in danger. Moreover, it is worth bearing in mind that many LGBT youth (28.4% in a recent survey)[9] have not disclosed their sexual minority orientation or transgender identity to either one or both of their parents. Some parents, however, may raise concerns about LGBT bullying to pediatricians. Pediatricians can encourage parents to regularly speak about bullying with their children to identify experiences of bullying and provide support if children are bullied. For example, parents can provide emotional support by emphasizing to youth that they do not deserve to be bullied. Pediatricians can also advise parents on how to report bullying to school officials and connect parents with resources on bullying. If bullying is not handled by school authorities, parents may be able to file a formal grievance with the US Department of Education's Office for Civil Rights and/or the US Department of Justice's Civil Rights Division.[49]

Pediatricians may engage in advocacy in their local schools and communities to address LGBT bullying. For example, pediatricians may voice support for enumerated laws that protect students from bullying and discrimination on the basis of sexual orientation and gender identity in states where they do not yet exist. They may also speak out against LGBT bullying to school officials and parents. Efforts to reduce LGBT bullying victimization should include addressing LGBT stigma in the broader community context. For example, physicians can advocate on behalf of transgender individuals by weighing in on bathroom use controversies in legislative hearings and amicus briefs.[7] LGBT bullying will likely persist as long as LGBT stigma exists within society.

DISCUSSION

LGBT bullying is prevalent among LGBT youth, with significant mental, behavioral, and physical health consequences. LGBT youth may be denied support from parents, teachers, and school administrators. Pediatricians therefore have a vital role to play in promoting the well-being of LGBT youth by preventing bullying, identifying bullying, offering counsel to youth who experience bullying and to their parents, and advocating for programs and policies to address LGBT bullying. Pediatricians have the power, ability, and responsibility to contribute to destigmatizing sexual and gender minority youth in their communities, thereby making the world a healthier place for their LGBT patients.

REFERENCES

1. Bolles A. Adam Kizer, bisexual teen, loses life by suicide after years of torment. GLAAD Web site. 2015. Available at: http://www.glaad.org/blog/adam-kizer-bisexual-teen-loses-life-suicide-after-years-torment. Accessed September 22, 2015.
2. Kellaway M. Subjected to 'constant' bullying, California trans teen dies by suicide. Advocate Web site. 2015. Available at: http://www.advocate.com/politics/transgender/2015/04/09/subjected-constant-bullying-california-trans-teen-dies-suicide. Accessed September 22, 2015.
3. Alesana T. Transgender Day of Remembrance. YouTube Web site. 2014. Available at: https://www.youtube.com/watch?v=F4H6wyUeVpE. Accessed September 22, 2015.
4. Alesana T. Acne!! YouTube Web site. 2015. Available at: https://www.youtube.com/watch?v=AtOsvoNSFxA. Accessed September 22, 2015.
5. Institute of Medicine (IOM). The health of lesbian, gay, bisexual, and transgender people: building a foundation for better understanding. Washington, DC: National Academies Press; 2011.
6. Ard KL, Makadon HJ. Improving the health care of lesbian, gay, bisexual and transgender (LGBT) people: understanding and eliminating health disparities. Boston: The Fenway Institute; Fenway Health; 2012.
7. Schuster MA, Reisner SL, Onorato SE. Beyond bathrooms – meeting the health needs of transgender people. N Engl J Med 2016;375:101–3.
8. Gladden RM, Vivolo-Kantor AM, Hamburger ME, et al. Bullying surveillance among youths: uniform definitions for public health and recommended data elements, version 1.0. Atlanta (GA): National Center for Injury Prevention and Control, Centers for Disease Control and Prevention and U.S. Department of Education; 2014.

9. Kosciw JG, Greytak EA, Bartkiewicz MJ, et al. The 2011 national school climate survey: the experiences of lesbian, gay, bisexual and transgender youth in our nation's schools. New York: Gay, Lesbian and Straight Education Network (GLSEN); 2012.

10. American Public Health Association. Reduction of bullying to address health disparities among LGBT Youth. Policy Statement 20142. Washington (DC): American Public Health Association; 2014.

11. Ybarra ML, Mitchell KJ, Palmer NA, et al. Online social support as a buffer against online and offline peer and sexual victimization among US LGBT and non-LGBT youth. Child Abuse Negl 2015;39:123–36.

12. Schuster MA, Bogart LM, Klein DJ, et al. A longitudinal study of bullying of sexual-minority youth. N Engl J Med 2015;372(19):1872–4.

13. Reisner SL, Greytak EA, Parsons JT, et al. Gender minority social stress in adolescence: Disparities in adolescent bullying and substance use by gender identity. J Sex Res 2015;52(3):243–56.

14. Swearer SM, Turner RK, Givens JE, et al. "You're so gay!": do different forms of bullying matter for adolescent males? School Psych Rev 2008;37(2):160.

15. Russell ST, Toomey RB, Ryan C, et al. Being out at school: the implications for school victimization and young adult adjustment. Amer J Orthopsych 2014; 84(6):635.

16. Russell ST, Everett BG, Rosario M, et al. Indicators of victimization and sexual orientation among adolescents: Analyses from Youth Risk Behavior Surveys. Am J Public Health 2014;104(2):255–61.

17. Hatzenbuehler ML, Duncan D, Johnson R. Neighborhood-level LGBT hate crimes and bullying among sexual minority youths: a geospatial analysis. Violence Vict 2015;30(4):663–75.

18. Poteat VP. Contextual and moderating effects of the peer group climate on use of homophobic epithets. School Psych Rev 2008;37(2):188.

19. Birkett M, Espelage DL. Homophobic name-calling, peer-groups, and masculinity: the socialization of homophobic behavior in adolescents. Soc Dev 2015;24(1): 184–205.

20. Poteat VP, DiGiovanni CD, Scheer JR. Predicting homophobic behavior among heterosexual youth: domain general and sexual orientation-specific factors at the individual and contextual level. J Youth Adolesc 2013;42(3):351–62.

21. Herek GM. Beyond "homophobia": thinking about sexual prejudice and stigma in the twenty-first century. Sex Res Soc Pol 2004;1(2):6–24.

22. Poteat VP, Anderson CJ. Developmental changes in sexual prejudice from early to late adolescence: the effects of gender, race, and ideology on different patterns of change. Devel Psych 2012;48(5):1403.

23. Friedman MS, Koeske GF, Silvestre AJ, et al. The impact of gender-role nonconforming behavior, bullying, and social support on suicidality among gay male youth. J Adol Health 2006;38(5):621–3.

24. Russell ST, Joyner K. Adolescent sexual orientation and suicide risk: Evidence from a national study. Am J Public Health 2001;91(8):1276–81.

25. Bogart LM, Elliott MN, Klein DJ, et al. Peer victimization in fifth grade and health in tenth grade. Pediatrics 2014;133(3):440–7.

26. Russell ST, Sinclair KO, Poteat VP, et al. Adolescent health and harassment based on discriminatory bias. Amer J Public Health 2012;102:493–5.

27. Díaz RM, Ayala G, Bein E. Sexual risk as an outcome of social oppression: Data from a probability sample of Latino gay men in three U.S. cities. Cultr Divers Ethnic Minor Psychol 2004;10:255–67.

28. Li MJ, DiStefano A, Mouttapa M, et al. Bias-motivated bullying and psychosocial problems: implications for HIV risk behaviors among young men who have sex with men. AIDS Care 2014;26(2):246–56.
29. Fekkes M. Do bullied children get ill, or do ill children get bullied? A Prospective cohort study on the relationship between bullying and health-related symptoms. Pediatrics 2006;117:1568–74.
30. Rosenthal L, Earnshaw VA, Carroll-Scott A, et al. Weight-and race-based bullying: Health associations among urban adolescents. J Health Psych 2015; 20(4):401–12.
31. Gini G, Pozzoli T. Association between bullying and psychosomatic problems: a meta-analysis. Pediatrics 2009;123(3):1059–65.
32. Gini G, Pozzoli T. Bullied children and psychosomatic problems: a meta-analysis. Pediatrics 2013;132(4):720–9.
33. Pascoe EA, Smart Richman L. Perceived discrimination and health: a meta-analytic review. Psych Bull 2009;135:531–54.
34. Birkett M, Newcomb ME, Mustanski B. Does it get better? A longitudinal analysis of psychological distress and victimization in lesbian, gay, bisexual, transgender, and questioning youth. J Adoles Health 2015;56(3):280–5.
35. Li MJ, DiStefano A, Mouttapa M, et al. Bias-motivated bullying and psychosocial problems: Implications for HIV risk behaviors among young men who have sex with men. AIDS Care 2014;26(2):246–56.
36. Roberts AL, Rosario M, Slopen N, et al. Childhood gender nonconformity, bullying victimization, and depressive symptoms across adolescence and early adulthood: An 11-year longitudinal study. J Am Acad Child Adol Psych 2013;52(2): 143–52.
37. Toomey RB, Ryan C, Diaz RM, et al. Gender-nonconforming lesbian, gay, bisexual, and transgender youth: School victimization and young adult psychosocial adjustment. Devel Psych 2010;46(6):1580.
38. Rivers I. Recollections of bullying at school and their long-term implications for lesbians, gay men, and bisexuals. Crisis 2004;25(4):169–75.
39. The Resilience Project. American Academy of Pediatrics Web site. Available at: https://www.aap.org/en-us/advocacy-and-policy/aap-health-initiatives/resilience/Pages/default.aspx. Accessed September 25, 2015.
40. LGBT Resources. American Medical Association Web site. Available at: http://www.ama-assn.org/ama/pub/about-ama/our-people/member-groups-sections/glbt-advisory-committee/glbt-resources.page? Accessed September 25, 2015.
41. Get Help Now. Stopbullying.gov Web site. Available at: http://www.stopbullying.gov/get-help-now/index.html. Accessed October 26, 2015.
42. Bullying and LGBT Youth. Stopbullying.gov Web site. Available at: http://www.stopbullying.gov/at-risk/groups/lgbt/index.html. Accessed October 27, 2015.
43. State Maps. GLSEN: Gay, Lesbian & Straight Education Network. Web site. Available at: https://www.glsen.org/article/state-maps. Accessed September 22, 2015.
44. Ali R. Dear colleague letter: sexual violence. Web site. 2011. Available at: https://www.whitehouse.gov/sites/default/files/dear_colleague_sexual_violence.pdf. Accessed September 22, 2015.
45. Schuster MA, Bogart LM. Did the ugly duckling have PTSD? Bullying, its effects, and the role of pediatricians. Pediatrics 2012;131:e288–91.
46. Glew G, Rivara F, Feudtner C. Bullying: children hurting children. Pediatrics Rev 2000;21(6):183–9.

47. Meckler GD, Elliott MN, Kanouse DE, et al. Nondisclosure of sexual orientation to a physician among a sample of gay, lesbian, and bisexual youth. Arch Pediatr Adolesc Med 2006;160(12):1248–54.

48. Marshall A, Yarber WL, Sherwood-Laughlin CM, et al. Coping and survival skills: The role school personnel play regarding support for bullied sexual minority-oriented youth. J School Health 2015;85(5):334–40.

49. Federal Laws. Stopbullying.gov Web site. 2014. Available at: http://www. stopbullying.gov/laws/federal/. Accessed September 22, 2015.

Lesbian, Gay, Bisexual, and Transgender Youth and Family Acceptance

 CrossMark

Sabra L. Katz-Wise, PhD[a,b,*], Margaret Rosario, PhD[c],
Michael Tsappis, MD[a,d,e]

KEYWORDS

- LGBT • Youth • Family • Support • Acceptance

KEY POINTS

- Parent–child attachment has implications for developing healthy relationships later in life.
- LGBT youth may experience a disruption in parent–child attachment if they are rejected based on their sexual orientation or gender identity.
- Parental rejection of LGBT youth negatively affects youths' identity and health.
- Parental acceptance of LGBT youth is crucial to ensure that youth develop a healthy sense of self.

INTRODUCTION

In this article, we discuss sexual minority, that is, lesbian, gay, and bisexual (LGB) and transgender (LGBT) youth. Sexual orientation refers to the individual's object of sexual or romantic attraction or desire, whether of the same or other sex relative to the individual's sex,[1] with sexual minority individuals having a sexual orientation that is partly or exclusively focused on the same sex. Transgender refers to individuals for whom current gender identity and sex assigned at birth are not concordant, whereas cisgender refers to individuals for whom current gender identity is congruent with sex assigned at birth.[1,2] Sexual orientation and gender identity are distinct aspects of the self. Transgender individuals may or may not be sexual minorities, and vice versa.

The authors have nothing to disclose.

[a] Division of Adolescent/Young Adult Medicine, Boston Children's Hospital, 300 Longwood Avenue, Boston, MA 02115, USA; [b] Department of Pediatrics, Harvard Medical School, 25 Shattuck St, Boston, MA 02115, USA; [c] Department of Psychology, City University of New York–City College and Graduate Center, 160 Convent Avenue, New York, NY 10031, USA; [d] Division of Psychiatry, Boston Children's Hospital, 300 Longwood Avenue, Boston, MA 02115, USA; [e] Department of Psychiatry, Harvard Medical School, Boston, MA, USA
* Corresponding author. Division of Adolescent/Young Adult Medicine, Boston Children's Hospital, 300 Longwood Avenue, Boston, MA 02115.
E-mail address: sabra.katz-wise@childrens.harvard.edu

Little is known about transgender youth, although some of the psychosocial experiences of cisgender sexual minority youth may generalize to this population.

The Institute of Medicine recently concluded that LGBT youth are at increased risk for poor mental and physical health compared with heterosexual and cisgender peers.[2] Indeed, representative samples of youth have found disparities by sexual orientation in health-related risk behaviors, symptomatology, and diagnoses,[3–8] with disparities persisting over time.[9–11] Furthermore, sexual orientation disparities exist regardless how sexual orientation is defined, whether by sexual or romantic attractions; sexual behaviors; self-identification as heterosexual, bisexual, lesbian/gay or other identities; or any combination thereof. Disparities by gender identity have also been found, with transgender youth experiencing poorer mental health than cisgender youth.[12]

Attempts have been made to understand sexual orientation and gender identity-related health disparities among youth. It has been argued that sexual minority youth experience stress associated with society's stigmatization of homosexuality and of anyone perceived to be homosexual (see Mark L. Hatzenbuehler and John E. Pachankis' article, "Stigma and Minority Stress as Social Determinants of Health Among LGBT Youth: Research Evidence and Clinical Implications," in this issue). This "gay-related"[13] or "minority" stress[14] is experienced at the hands of others as victimization. It is also internalized, such that sexual minorities victimize the self by means, for example, of possessing negative attitudes toward homosexuality, known as internalized homonegativity or homophobia. In addition to interpersonal stigma and internalized stigma, the main focus of this article, structural stigma reflected in societal-level norms, policies, and laws also play a significant role in sexual minority stress, and is discussed in Mark L. Hatzenbuehler and John E. Pachankis' article, "Stigma and Minority Stress as Social Determinants of Health Among LGBT Youth: Research Evidence and Clinical Implications," in this issue. Meta-analytic reviews find that sexual minorities experience more stress relative to heterosexuals, as well as unique stressors.[6,15,16] Research also indicates that transgender individuals experience substantial amounts of prejudice, discrimination, and victimization,[17] and are thought to experience a similar process of minority stress as experienced by sexual minorities,[18] although minority stress for transgender individuals is based primarily on stigma related to gender identity rather than stigma related to having a minority sexual orientation. Stigma related to gender expression affects those with gender nonconforming behavior, a group that includes both transgender and cisgender individuals. This includes many cisgender youth growing up with LGB orientations.

Actual or anticipated family acceptance or rejection of LGBT youth is important in understanding the youth's experience of minority stress, how the youth is likely to cope with the stress, and, consequently, the impact of minority stress on the youth's health.[19] This article addresses the role of family, in particular parental acceptance and rejection in LGBT youths' identity and health. Literature reviewed in this article focuses on the experiences of sexual minority cisgender youth owing to a lack of research on transgender youth. However, we include findings and implications for transgender youth whenever possible.

THEORIES OF PARENTAL ACCEPTANCE AND REJECTION

The continued importance of parents in the lives of youth is indisputable: beginning at birth, extending through adolescence, and even into emerging adulthood, affecting all relationships beyond those with the parents, and determining the individual's own sense of self-worth. Attachment accounts for this vast reach and influence of parents.

According to Bowlby,[20–22] attachment to the primary caretaker guarantees survival because the attachment system is activated during stress and concerns the accessibility and responsiveness of the attachment figure to the child's distress and potential danger. The pattern or style of attachment that develops is based on repeated interactions or transactions with the primary caregiver during infancy and childhood. Those experiences, in interaction with constitutional factors like temperament, influence the internal working model (ie, mental representations of emotion, behavior, and thought) of beliefs about and expectations concerning the accessibility and responsiveness of the attachment figure. In time, this internal working model influences perceptions of others, significantly influencing patterns in relationships over time and across settings. The beliefs and expectations concerning the attachment figure also affect the internal working model of the self, meaning the individual's sense of self-worth.

The 3 consistent patterns of attachment that arise in infancy and childhood are related to the internal working models of the self and other. The "secure" child has positive models of the self and other because the primary attachment figure has been accessible when needed and responsive in an attuned and sensitive manner to the child's needs and capabilities. Consequently, the securely attached child is able to regulate emotion, explore the environment, and become self-reliant in an age-appropriate manner. The "insecure" child has an inaccessible and unresponsive primary caregiver, who is intrusive, erratic, or abusive. One of 2 insecure attachment patterns emerges. In the first pattern, the child dismisses or avoids the parent, becoming "compulsively"[21] self-reliant and regulating emotion even when contraindicated. This child with "avoidant/dismissive" attachment depends on the self, possessing a positive internal working model of the self but a negative one of the other. In the second insecure attachment pattern, the child is anxiously preoccupied with the caregiver but in a resistant (ie, distressed or aroused) manner. The individual with "anxious/preoccupied/resistant/ambivalent" attachment has a negative working model of the self, but a positive model of the other.

Attachment patterns in childhood are partly related to character traits in adulthood, and have implications for emotion regulation from the perspective of coping with stress, as detailed elsewhere.[23,24] Based on positive working models of the self and other, the securely attached individual approaches a stressful situation in an adaptive manner that allows for a realistic appraisal of the situation and a selection of coping strategies most likely to reduce or eliminate the stressor or, at minimum, render the stressor tolerable. By comparison, insecurely attached individuals may distort reality because they may be more likely to appraise a situation as stressful, even when it is not. They may also be maladaptive in their management of stress and use emotion-focused coping strategies, such as substance use, to improve mood and tolerate stress. These patterns of coping influenced by attachment are present by and common in adolescence.[25] Coping is critical because sexual orientation and gender development are potentially stressful experiences for all youth, but especially for sexual and gender minorities, given the frequent stigmatization of homosexuality, gender nonconforming behavior, and gender-variant identities.[19]

IMPLICATIONS FOR PARENT–CHILD ATTACHMENT

The vast majority of sexual minority youth are born to heterosexual parents. Those parents may not uncommonly possess implicit or explicit negative attitudes toward homosexuality and expect their children to be heterosexual. Parents may not only be surprised that their child may be or is a sexual minority, but they may also respond negatively to the child. Similarly, the vast majority of transgender and/or gender nonconforming youth are born to cisgender and/or gender conforming parents, who often possess negative attitudes toward those who violate societal expectations for gender identity, expression, and roles, and expect their children to be cisgender and gender conforming. Negative responses from parents to LGBT youth may range from anxious concerns about the child's well-being and future to abuse and even banishment of the child from the home.

The range of possible parental responses to the child's sexual orientation, gender-related behavior, or identity when these deviate from parental expectation is linked to the child's attachment.[24] The securely attached youth has parents who have encouraged age-appropriate exploration and value the child as a unique individual. Such parents may be surprised and concerned by the child's sexual minority orientation, gender nonconformity, or transgender identity, but they are likely to work through their negative attitudes over time and continue to be accessible and responsive to their child. Thus, the attachment of the securely attached youth may be shaken when parents learn of these, but it is unlikely to be undone. This does not apply to insecurely attached youth, given their a priori inaccessible, unresponsive, and potentially abusive parents. Knowledge of these deviations from expectation, coupled with negative attitudes, may lead such parents to be less supportive of their child, or reject them. The latter may manifest in parental abuse of the youth, running away by the youth to escape maltreatment, or eviction of the youth from the home.

Representative samples of youth find that, relative to heterosexual peers, sexual minorities report lower levels of parental closeness[26] and increased rates of parental abuse[6,27] and homelessness.[28–32] Transgender youth also report elevated rates of child abuse[13] compared with their cisgender peers. More specifically, sexual minority youth relative to heterosexual peers and siblings report less secure attachment to their mothers and their mothers report less affection for them.[33] It has also been found that maternal attachment mediates sexual orientation disparities in depressive symptomatology and substance use.[33,34] These disparities in sexual and gender minority youth from their gender normative peers and siblings involving the degree of attachment underscore the importance of parental attitudes toward sexual minority orientations, gender-nonconforming behavior, and gender identity variance for secure attachment in youth. Pediatric clinicians should assess these and the quality of the parent–child attachment.

These attachment implications and findings take on added meaning when considered along with youth's neurocognitive development and coping capabilities. It is known that development of the prefrontal cortex lags behind that of limbic regions during adolescence,[35] ensuring less impulse control and greater risk taking.[36] The findings extend to emotion regulation. Human imaging studies demonstrate that youth have a difficult time downregulating amygdala activation.[37] Therefore, coping in youth is circumscribed by limited ability to rationally or logically plan, execute, evaluate, and readjust a problem-focused strategy to eliminate or reduce stress, while simultaneously controlling emotional reactivity.

Consequently, youth greatly depend on adults, especially parents, both to assist them with meeting developmental demands and to guide their personal experiences in various domains (eg, interpersonal, romantic) and settings (eg, school, work). LGBT youth with insecure attachment may have a difficult time navigating and coping with such challenges if their parents are inaccessible and unresponsive.

Nevertheless, attachment may change over time.[38] This may happen if the attachment figure becomes more or less accessible and responsive, or if 1 attachment figure (eg, the mother) buffers the negative impact of another attachment figure (eg, the father). A nonparental individual may provide support, but whether she or he can provide the deep sense of security and the safe haven of an attachment figure is uncertain, particularly if social structures and cultural traditions do not foster these relationships.

Parental Reactions to Gender Nonconformity

Gender nonconformity, defined as having a gender expression that is perceived to be inconsistent with gender norms expected for an individual's sex,[39] is not uncommon in children. A study of gender atypical behavior (1 aspect of gender nonconformity) among elementary school children found that approximately 23% of boys and 39% of girls displayed multiple gender atypical behaviors.[40] Gender nonconformity exists on a spectrum, with some children displaying less and some children displaying more gender nonconformity. This spectrum has implications for victimization, such that youth who are more gender nonconforming are at increased risk for abuse by caregivers,[41] as well as peer victimization and bullying (see Valerie A. Earnshaw and colleagues' article, "Bullying among Lesbian, Gay, Bisexual, and Transgender Youth," in this issue) and an increased risk of depressive symptoms.[42] Although a link exists between childhood gender nonconformity and later sexual minority orientation[43] and/or transgender identity,[44] not all children who are gender nonconforming are LGB or transgender in later adolescence or adulthood.[44]

As with stigma attached to sexual minorities and transgender individuals, gender nonconformity is also stigmatized in and of itself, particularly among boys. Connell's theory of hegemonic masculinity sheds light on this stigma; it suggests that 1 form of masculinity, with features such as aggression, limited emotionality, and heterosexuality, is culturally exalted above others.[45,46] For this reason, variation from this level of masculinity among boys can be stigmatized. Similar to stigma related to sexual minorities and transgender individuals, stigma related to gender nonconformity is often enacted through prejudice, discrimination, and victimization. A study of early adolescents found that gender nonconformity was associated with increased victimization by peers.[47] Youth who are sexual minorities may be bullied for gender nonconformity before they are aware of their sexual orientation. A recent study found that sexual minority youth were bullied as early as fifth grade, which is before the majority of sexual minority youth are aware of their sexual orientation or disclose it to others.[48] Although the study did not assess the reason for bullying, it is possible that these youth were bullied based on gender nonconformity.

Negative societal views may include adverse parental reactions to a child's gender nonconformity. A qualitative study found that parents welcomed gender nonconformity among their daughters, but had mixed reactions to their sons' gender nonconformity; they accepted some level of nonconformity in their sons (eg, interest in cooking), but had negative reactions to higher levels of nonconformity (eg, wearing dresses).[49] In addition to increased risk for bullying victimization from peers, previous research has found that gender nonconforming children have a high prevalence of childhood sexual abuse, physical abuse, and psychological abuse by caregivers,[41,50] which may be indicative of negative parental reactions to their child's gender nonconformity. Parents' initial reactions to gender nonconformity in their children may extend to reactions to youth's sexual orientation disclosure.

PARENTAL REACTIONS TO YOUTHS' LESBIAN, GAY, BISEXUAL, AND TRANSGENDER DISCLOSURE

Disclosure of sexual orientation to family members is common among sexual minority youth. One study found that 79% of sexual minority youth had disclosed their sexual orientation to at least 1 parent, and two-thirds of youth had disclosed their orientation to at least 1 sibling and 1 extended family member.[51] Another study of sexual minority emerging adults found that 46% of men and 44% of women had disclosed their sexual orientation to their parents.[52] In this study, participants were more likely to disclose their sexual orientation to their mothers than to their fathers, and disclosures typically occurred around age 19 years in a face-to-face encounter.

A number of theories have been proposed to conceptualize the reactions of parents to their children's disclosure of sexual minority orientation,[53] including mourning/loss paradigms based on Kubler-Ross's stage model of grief[54] and family stress theory.[55,56] Willoughby and colleagues applied family stress theory to parental reactions to their children's sexual orientation disclosure, proposing that reactions may depend on the availability of family-level resources (eg, relational competencies)[57,58] to manage stress, meanings that parents attributed to the stressful event (eg, believing that sexual orientation is a choice), and cooccurring stressors (eg, divorce, major illness).[59] Although these theories are useful for understanding parents' reactions to their child's sexual orientation disclosure, some researchers have proposed that these models are limited in that they may not describe the reaction of all parents, account for developmental change in reactions over time, or consider the experiences of the child.[53]

Parents may experience a number of different responses when faced with a disclosure of sexual minority orientation from their child, ranging from accepting to rejecting. Research in this area has yielded mixed results regarding the positivity and negativity of parental reactions. One study found that sexual minority youth who had disclosed their sexual orientation to family members reported more verbal and physical abuse by family members and more suicidality compared with youth who had not disclosed their orientation.[60] However, this study was published in 1998 and much has changed since then regarding societal acceptance of sexual minorities. Another study found that, among sexual minority youth who had disclosed their sexual orientation to their mother or father, the majority (89%–97%) received a positive reaction.[61] However, these findings may be misleading, given they do not consider how many youth have not disclosed to parents owing to fear of negative reactions or rejection.

A review of the sexual minority literature finds that one-third of youth experience parental acceptance, another one-third experience parental rejection, and the remaining one-third do not disclose their sexual orientation, even by their late teenage years and early 20s.[19] The review also finds that regardless of initial reactions, parents generally become more accepting of their child over time. For instance, 1 study found that, compared with sexual minority youth who had not disclosed their sexual orientation to parents, sexual minority youth who had disclosed their orientation reported more past sexual orientation-based verbal victimization from parents, but more current family support and less fear of future parental victimization,[62] indicating greater acceptance over time. Whether such findings generalize to transgender youth is unknown. Our first case vignette in this article illustrates areas needing more empirical research regarding transgender youth's disclosure of gender identity to parents (**Box 1**).

The process of sexual orientation disclosure in families may be shaped by the values of the family system.[63] In 1 study investigating traditional values and family acceptance of sexual minorities, families with a strong emphasis on traditional values (eg, importance of religion, emphasis on marriage, emphasis on having children) were perceived as less accepting of sexual minority orientation than less traditional families.[64] Parental responses to youth's disclosure of sexual minority orientation may also differ based on race/ethnicity or cultural levels of acceptance of sexual

Box 1
Case 1

A 16 year-old natal male presented to the physician with his mother and father with a chief complaint of depression. He reported feelings of worthlessness, failure, unhappiness, and becoming easily overwhelmed and emotionally numb when stressed. During that first meeting he made a point of reporting that he had grown to feel more distant from his mother and father.

A referral was made for individual psychotherapy. During subsequent follow-up appointments, the depressive symptoms remained unchanged. There was ongoing resistance to therapy but during the course of care a positive alliance was developed with the physician. It was noted later in the treatment that the physician's neutral, inquisitive style, appearance of nonjudgment and of agency for the patient, and signaling of a primary alliance with the patient rather than the parents (while maintaining respect for the parents' interests), all helped to establish a good clinical alliance with the patient.

Seven months into the treatment relationship, an appointment was scheduled with the physician at the patient's request. The stated goal for the meeting was to inform the physician, "I'm a girl. I don't feel like I'm a girl, I *am* a girl." The patient reported constant preoccupation with thoughts related to their current gender identity, efforts to cope with already developed secondary sex characteristics, and how to achieve gender affirmation. The patient indicated a preference for the use of feminine gender pronouns. The patient also chose to come out to her mother in the office with the physician present. Her mother was able to express an interest in understanding what was being explained to her but anticipated a slow process. The patient left the office indicating that the mother's response was consistent with her [the patient's] expectations.

The next scheduled appointment occurred 2 weeks later. By that time the patient had told her father, who did not attend the visit. Her father's response was experienced as reserved and without clear acceptance or rejection. The drive to come out seemed to have been amplified since the initial experience with her mother. Beginning with a trusted faculty counselor at school and then with teachers and finally peers, she had informed members of her school and social community about her gender identity. The patient experienced their responses as supportive. There were no reports of explicit or implicit mistreatment. Her parents remained avoidant, however.

The patient felt an urgent drive to take action in the period after gender identity disclosure. After informing her broader social community, the patient sought to formally change her name and remained focused on gender affirmation. The family rejected the psychotherapist's suggestion to consult with a gender management service, saying they would not agree to this "until [he's] 18."

The patient's symptoms of depression continued, despite apparent relief and transient mood improvement immediately after the initial gender identity disclosure. Because depression returned after her mother's and then father's avoidant responses, the patient seemed to be driven to repeat the disclosure to an expanding set of her social community. Each supportive encounter resulted in another transient improvement in mood, but these were always followed by recurrence of depression. Observing and discussing that process with the patient led to a calming of the fervent drive to act, but the depression remained. The patient eventually abandoned efforts to obtain a supportive and accepting response from her parents, and elected to defer pursuing further gender affirmation until able to do so independently, including suspending social transition, such as requesting to be addressed by feminine name and pronoun. The depression was ultimately treated with antidepressant medication.

minority individuals (see Errol Fields and colleagues' article, "The intersection of sociocultural factors and health-related behavior in LGBT youth: experiences among young black gay males as an example," in this issue). However, only 1 study, as far as we know, has examined parental responses to youths' sexual orientation disclosure by race/ethnicity among young adult gay males of African American, European–American, Mexican–American, and Vietnamese–American backgrounds. It found family responses to be similar across the 4 groups.[63]

Additional research on levels of family support and rejection of sexual minority youth has found group differences by sexual orientation, race/ethnicity, and gender. A study of sexual orientation group differences in parental support of young adults found that lesbian and bisexual women reported lower levels of parental support than heterosexual women, and that gay men reported lower levels of parental support than bisexual or heterosexual men.[65] These group differences may be related to general attitudes toward different sexual orientation groups, indicating that attitudes toward sexual minority individuals are more negative than attitudes toward heterosexual individuals.[66] Some race/ethnicity differences in level of family support have also been found. In a study of White and Latino sexual minority young adults, Latino men reported the highest number of negative family reactions to their sexual orientation in adolescence.[67] However, another study found similar levels of parental support among WHITE and racial/ethnic minority LGBT youth.[68] More research is needed to obtain a clearer picture of how race/ethnicity may be related to parental responses to sexual orientation disclosure among youth, as well as parental support and rejection of LGBT youth (see Errol Fields and colleagues' article, "The intersection of sociocultural factors and health-related behavior in LGBT youth: experiences among young black gay males as an example," in this issue for more information). Although there is little research on family support and rejection of transgender youth, some research has indicated that these youth report more rejection than cisgender youth.[69] Further empirical research is needed to investigate family support and rejection among transgender youth, particularly compared with cisgender sexual minority youth.

IMPLICATIONS FOR LESBIAN, GAY, BISEXUAL, AND TRANSGENDER YOUTH IDENTITY AND HEALTH

Levels of family acceptance and rejection may have implications for the identity development of sexual minority youth. A study of sexual minority adolescents and young adults examined associations between parental acceptance and identity profiles that were affirmed as opposed to being characterized by struggle.[70] Results indicated that less parental rejection was associated with a greater likelihood of having an affirmed identity than struggling with one's identity,[70] suggesting that the level of parental rejection may affect youths' ability to accept their own sexual minority identity. Similarly, youth whose parents knew about their sexual orientation reported less "internalized homophobia" (or self-stigma; see Mark L. Hatzenbuehler and John E. Pachankis' article, "Stigma and Minority Stress as Social Determinants of Health Among LGBT Youth: Research Evidence and Clinical Implications," in this issue) compared both with youth whose parents did not know about their sexual orientation and youth who newly disclosed their orientation to their parents over the course of the study.[71]

Pediatric care providers should be aware that family rejection may have serious consequences for the physical and mental health of LGBT youth.[67,72] Studies have found that parental rejection is associated with health risk behaviors and poor mental and physical health outcomes among LGBT individuals. Sexual minority emerging adults with higher levels of family rejection were more likely to report attempted suicide, high levels of depression, and illegal drug use, and engagement in unprotected sexual intercourse.[67] Parental rejection negatively affects health among both transgender and cisgender adolescents. In the Thai study referenced earlier, family rejection predicted adolescents' level of depression, suicidal thinking, and sexual risk behaviors among both transgender and cisgender youth.[69]

Conversely, family acceptance may be protective for LGBT youth's health. Among sexual minority youth, adolescents whose mothers responded positively to their sexual orientation disclosure were less likely to use substances compared with those who had not disclosed their orientation to their parents or whose mothers and fathers did not react positively.[61] In addition, family support and acceptance is associated with greater self-esteem, social support, and general health status, as well as less depression, less substance abuse, and less suicidal ideation and behaviors among LGBT youth.[72] Family support is also associated with less substance use among LGBT youth.[72–74] Among transgender youth specifically, parental support is protective against depression[75] and associated with having a better quality of life.[75]

CLINICAL IMPLICATIONS

The preceding information underscores why it is important for providers of pediatric care to know the effects of family nonacceptance and rejection on youth; to understand specific threats to family acceptance affecting LGBT youth like parental stigma against LGB orientation, gender nonconforming behavior, and/or transgender identities; to assess these in youth and families; and to intervene appropriately in case of family nonacceptance or risk for it. The following case vignettes illustrate these principles in clinical practice.

Case 1 (see **Box 1**) illustrates several complexities of coming out as transgender during the later adolescent period. The burden of unshared personal information and associated shame and fears of rejection, especially by one's closest supports, combined with the mental effort required to maintain an external identity at odds with the internal sense of true self all contributed significantly to this patient's depression. Improvement in depression was observed with disclosure to the mother, but depression recurred after subsequent negative or ambivalent parental responses. Acceptance was achieved within a broader social network, but peer and other community support could not replace the desired parental reaction. Without the support of the parents, the patient regressed and acquiesced to the sex assigned at birth, followed by depression that required pharmacologic treatment. Although the pediatrician and psychotherapist were not able to effect parental acceptance, treatment was used to clarify its importance as a way to set the stage for further family work or adaptive separation, individuation, and coping with ongoing family nonacceptance.

In Case 2 (**Box 2**), the child benefited from the protective effects of supportive parents to whom she seemed to have a secure attachment. Her masculine gender expression provoked mistreatment from peers. The stress of her exclusion began to affect her psychological health, but was modified by her ability to share her feelings and experiences at school with her parents and to rely on their ability to provide support and take appropriate protective action. A good relationship with the pediatrician extended the foundation of support. Together they were able to care for the child through an environmental action that may have prevented the need for mental health care. This case also underscores that gender nonconforming behavior may, but does not necessarily, mean that the youth will have an LGB orientation or be transgender later in adolescence or adulthood.

Box 2
Case 2

The pediatrician had provided primary care for a girl since her birth. She experienced an unremarkable early development and had remained medically healthy. She was clearly "a tomboy" as her mom would note, but this garnered no concern as it might if instead of a masculine girl she were a feminine boy. There was no interest in dolls or princesses, no comfort in wearing a dress, and no affinity for pink or purple. She wore jeans and T-shirts, played football with the boys at recess, and was comfortable getting dirty.

During her fourth grade year, a Monday office visit was scheduled after an episode of emesis at school. Her mother explained that the previous week, her daughter had been complaining of stomachaches and headaches in the morning. She had stayed home from school on Friday, but seemed better by that afternoon and over the weekend. On Monday morning she had again complained of feeling sick. Her examination was unremarkable. Physically she was well. Reassurance was given along with written authorization to return to school the next day.

School avoidance continued. Given the doctor's findings, she was not kept home. She began to pick at her skin and seemed to be unhappy. Her parents had always been caring and attentive though not intrusive. They asked what had been happening at school. Their daughter explained that a bully had called her "gay" and said she was "a lesbian." In the absence of effective intervention for bullying by her school, her persistent masculine gender expression elicited name-calling by a bully, which led to a group dynamic of teasing by other children at school. This led to widespread peer rejection and shunning. Her parents listened and supported her. A meeting was arranged at the school where the teacher acknowledged awareness of recent shifts in friendships. Although he and school administration acknowledged the problem, they did not implement standard antibullying interventions (see Valerie A. Earnshaw and colleagues' article, "Bullying among Lesbian, Gay, Bisexual, and Transgender Youth," in this issue), expressing confidence that the peer ostracism would pass quickly without school intervention.

However, peer perceptions of her sexual orientation and associated social ostracism did not change. With her parents' support and encouragement, she was able to attend school. Her skin picking resolved, but she remained unhappy. After speaking with their daughter, the parents requested a school district transfer, but were opposed by school administration.

Parents sought help from the pediatrician, asking for a letter of medical necessity. The pediatrician readily provided one that included information about negative health effects of bullying, social isolation, and alienation resulting from gender nonconformity and perceived sexual minority status. She included information about increased risk of depression and suicide. After receiving the letter, the school district approved a transfer.

Adjustment to the new school, which had an antibullying policy and curriculum that included nontolerance of bullying on the basis of sexual orientation and gender, was positive. The patient's mood improved quickly after the transfer. She found friends who introduced her to a new hobby of freestyle skateboarding. Now a teenager, she has become quite accomplished. Both she and her current boyfriend participate in the same competitive skateboard circuit.

SUMMARY

In this article, we have discussed theories of attachment, parental acceptance and rejection, and implications of each for LGBT youths' identity and health. We have provided 2 clinical cases to illustrate the impact of family acceptance and rejection of a transgender youth and a gender nonconforming youth who was neither a sexual minority nor transgender. It is clear from existing research that family acceptance and rejection is crucial to the health and well-being of LGBT youth. However, the majority of research conducted in this area has focused on sexual minority cisgender youth. More research is needed to understand how family acceptance and rejection affects the health of transgender and gender nonconforming youth. Health care providers working with LGBT youth should address issues of family acceptance and rejection during clinical visits to ensure that youth develop a healthy sense of self in terms of their sexual orientation and gender identity.

REFERENCES

1. Rosario M, Schrimshaw EW. Theories and etiologies of sexual orientation. In: Tolman DL, Diamond LM, editors. APA handbook of sexuality and psychology. Washington, DC: American Psychological Association; 2014. p. 555–96.
2. Institute of Medicine. The health of lesbian, gay, bisexual, and transgender people: building a foundation for better understanding. Washington, DC: The National Academies Press; 2011.
3. Austin SB, Nelson LA, Birkett MA, et al. Eating disorder symptoms and obesity at the intersections of gender, ethnicity, and sexual orientation in US high school students. Am J Public Health 2013;103(2):e16–22.
4. Fergusson DM, Horwood LJ, Beautrais AL. Is sexual orientation related to mental health problems and suicidality in young people? Arch Gen Psychiatry 1999; 56(10):876–80. Available at: http://www.ncbi.nlm.nih.gov/pubmed/10530626. Accessed October 10, 2015.
5. Marshal MP, Friedman MS, Stall R, et al. Sexual orientation and adolescent substance use: a meta-analysis and methodological review. Addiction 2008;103(4): 546–56.
6. Friedman MS, Marshal MP, Guadamuz TE, et al. A meta-analysis of disparities in childhood sexual abuse, parental physical abuse, and peer victimization among sexual minority and sexual nonminority individuals. Am J Public Health 2011; 101(8):1481–94.
7. Rosario M, Corliss HL, Everett BG, et al. Sexual orientation disparities in cancer-related risk behaviors of tobacco, alcohol, sexual behaviors, and diet and physical activity: pooled Youth Risk Behavior Surveys. Am J Public Health 2014; 104(2):245–54.
8. Wichstrøm L. Sexual orientation as a risk factor for bulimic symptoms. Int J Eat Disord 2006;39(6):448–53.
9. Marshal MP, Friedman MS, Stall R, Thompson AL. Individual trajectories of substance use in lesbian, gay and bisexual youth and heterosexual youth. Addiction 2009;104(6):974–81.
10. Needham BL. Sexual attraction and trajectories of mental health and substance use during the transition from adolescence to adulthood. J Youth Adolesc 2012; 41(2):179–90.
11. Rosario M, Li F, Wypij D, et al. Disparities by sexual orientation in frequent engagement in cancer-related risk behaviors: a 12-year follow-up. Am J Public Health 2016;106(4):698–706.
12. Reisner SL, Vetters R, Leclerc M, et al. Mental health of transgender youth in care at an adolescent urban community health center: a matched retrospective cohort study. J Adolesc Health 2015;56:274–9.
13. Rosario M, Schrimshaw EW, Hunter J, Gwadz M. Gay-related stress and emotional distress among gay, lesbian, and bisexual youths: a longitudinal examination. J Consult Clin Psychol 2002;70(4):967–75.
14. Meyer IH. Prejudice, social stress, and mental health in lesbian, gay, and bisexual populations: conceptual issues and research evidence. Psychol Bull 2003; 129(5):674–97.

15. Katz-Wise SL, Hyde JS. Victimization experiences of lesbian, gay, and bisexual individuals: a meta-analysis. J Sex Res 2012;49(2–3):142–67.

16. Newcomb ME, Mustanski B. Internalized homophobia and internalizing mental health problems: a meta-analytic review. Clin Psychol Rev 2010;30(8):1019–29.

17. Grant JM, Mottet LA, Tanis J, et al. Injustice at every turn: a report of the national transgender discrimination survey. 2011. Available at: http://www.thetaskforce.org/static_html/downloads/reports/reports/ntds_full.pdf.

18. Hendricks ML, Testa RJ. A conceptual framework for clinical work with transgender and gender nonconforming clients: an adaptation of the minority stress model. Prof Psychol Res Pract 2012;43(5):460–7.

19. Rosario M, Schrimshaw EW. The sexual identity development and health of lesbian, gay, and bisexual adolescents: an ecological perspective. In: Patterson CJ, D'Augelli AR, editors. Handbook of psychology and sexual orientation. New York: Oxford University Press; 2013. p. 87–101.

20. Bowlby J. Attachment and loss: volume I. Attachment. 2nd edition. New York: Basic Books; 1969.

21. Bowlby J. Attachment and loss: volume II. Separation: anxiety and anger. New York: Basic Books; 1973.

22. Bowlby J. Attachment and loss: volume III: loss: sadness and depression. New York: Basic Books; 1980.

23. Mikulincer M, Shaver PR. Attachment in adulthood: structure, dynamics, and change. New York: Guilford Press; 2007.

24. Rosario M. Implications of childhood experiences for the health and adaptation of lesbian, gay, and bisexual individuals: sensitivity to developmental process in future research. Psychol Sex Orientat Gend Divers 2015;2(3):214–24.

25. Seiffge-Krenke I. Coping with relationship stressors: the impact of different working models of attachment and links to adaptation. J Youth Adolesc 2006;35:25–39.

26. Pearson J, Wilkinson L. Family relationships and adolescent well-being: are families equally protective for same-sex attracted youth? J Youth Adolesc 2013;42(3):376–93.

27. Corliss HL, Cochran SD, Mays VM. Reports of parental maltreatment during childhood in a United States population-based survey of homosexual, bisexual, and heterosexual adults. Child Abuse Negl 2002;26:1165–78.

28. Corliss HL, Goodenow CS, Nichols L, et al. High burden of homelessness among sexual-minority adolescents: findings from a representative Massachusetts high school sample. Am J Public Health 2011;101(9):1683–9.

29. McLaughlin KA, Hatzenbuehler ML, Xuan Z, et al. Disproportionate exposure to early-life adversity and sexual orientation disparities in psychiatric morbidity. Child Abuse Negl 2012;36(9):645–55.

30. Rice E, Barman-Adhikari A, Rhoades H, et al. Homelessness experiences, sexual orientation, and sexual risk taking among high school students in Los Angeles. J Adolesc Health 2013;52(6):773–8.

31. Cashman SB, Allen AJ, Corburn J, et al. Analyzing and interpreting data with communities. In: Minkler M, Wallerstein N, editors. Community-based participatory research for health: From process to outcomes (2nd ed.). Analyzing and interpreting data with communities. San Francisco (CA): Jossey-Bass; 2008. p. 285–306.

32. Waller MW, Sanchez RP. The association between same-sex romantic attractions and relationships and running away among a nationally representative sample of adolescents. Child Adolesc Soc Work J 2011;28:475–93.

33. Rosario M, Reisner SL, Corliss HL, et al. Disparities in depressive distress by sexual orientation in emerging adults: the roles of attachment and stress paradigms. Arch Sex Behav 2014;43(5):901–16.

34. Rosario M, Reisner SL, Corliss HL, et al. Sexual-orientation disparities in substance use in emerging adults: a function of stress and attachment paradigms. Psychol Addict Behav 2014;28(3):790–804.
35. Casey BJ, Getz S, Galvan A. The adolescent brain. Dev Rev 2008;28(1):62–77.
36. Galvan A, Hare TA, Parra CE, et al. Earlier development of the accumbens relative to orbitofrontal cortex might underlie risk-taking behavior in adolescents. J Neurosci 2006;26(25):6885–92.
37. Hare TA, Tottenham N, Galvan A, et al. Biological substrates of emotional reactivity and regulation in adolescence during an emotional go-nogo task. Biol Psychiatry 2008;63(10):927–34.
38. Booth-LaForce C, Groh AM, Burchinal MR, et al. V. Caregiving and contextual sources of continuity and change in attachment security from infancy to late adolescence. Monogr Soc Res Child Dev 2014;79(3):67–84.
39. Green E, Maurer L. The teaching transgender toolkit: a Facilitator's guide to increasing knowledge, decreasing prejudice and building skills. Ithaca (NY): Planned Parenthood of the Southern Finger Lakes; 2015.
40. Sandberg DE, Meyer-Bahlburg HF, Ehrhardt AA, et al. The prevalence of gender-atypical behavior in elementary school children. J Am Acad Child Adolesc Psychiatry 1993;32(2):306–14.
41. Roberts AL, Rosario M, Corliss HL, et al. Childhood gender nonconformity: a risk indicator for childhood abuse and posttraumatic stress in youth. Pediatrics 2012; 129(3):410–7.
42. Roberts AL, Rosario M, Slopen N, et al. Childhood gender nonconformity, bullying victimization, and depressive symptoms across adolescence and early adulthood: an 11-year longitudinal study. J Am Acad Child Adolesc Psychiatry 2013;52(2):143–52.
43. Rieger G, Linsenmeier JAW, Gygax L, et al. Sexual orientation and childhood gender nonconformity: evidence from home videos. Dev Psychol 2008;44(1):46–58.
44. Wallien MS, Cohen-Kettenis PT. Psychosexual outcome of gender-dysphoric children. J Am Acad Child Adolesc Psychiatry 2008;47(12):1413–23.
45. Connell RW. Gender and power. Stanford (CA): Stanford University Press; 1987.
46. Connell RW. Masculinities. Berkeley (CA): University of California Press; 1995.
47. Aspenlieder L, Buchanan CM, McDougall P, et al. Gender nonconformity and peer victimization in pre- and early adolescence. Eur J Dev Sci 2009;3(1):3–16. Available at: http://ezp-prod1.hul.harvard.edu/login?url=http://search.ebscohost.com/login.aspx?direct=true&db=psyh&AN=2010-11950-002&site=ehost-live&scope=site.
48. Schuster MA, Bogart LM, Elliott MN. A longitudinal study of bullying of sexual-minority youth. N Engl J Med 2015;372:1872–4. Available at: http://www.nejm.org.ezp-prod1.hul.harvard.edu/doi/full/10.1056/NEJMc1413064. Accessed February 29, 2016.
49. Kane EW. "No way my boys are going to be like that!": parents' responses to children's gender nonconformity. Gend Soc 2006;20(2):149–76.
50. Roberts AL, Rosario M, Corliss HL, et al. Elevated risk of posttraumatic stress in sexual minority youths: mediation by childhood abuse and gender nonconformity. Am J Public Health 2012;102(8):1587–93.
51. Rosario M, Schrimshaw EW, Hunter J. Disclosure of sexual orientation and subsequent substance use and abuse among lesbian, gay, and bisexual youths: critical role of disclosure reactions. Psychol Addict Behav 2009;23(1):175–84.
52. Savin-Williams RC, Ream GL. Sex variations in the disclosure to parents of same-sex attractions. J Fam Psychol 2003;17(3):429–38.

53. Savin-Williams RC, Dube EM. Parental reactions to their child's disclosure of a gay/lesbian identity. Fam Relat 1998;47(1):7–13.

54. Kubler-Ross E. On death and dying. New York: MacMillan; 1969.

55. Hill R. Families under stress. Westport (CT): Greenwood; 1949.

56. McCubbin HI, Patterson JM. The family stress process: the double ABCX model of adjustment and adaptation. Marriage Fam Rev 1983;6:7–37.

57. McCubbin HI, Thompson AI, McCubbin MA. Family assessment: resiliency, coping and adaptation: inventories for research and practice. Madison (WI): University of Wisconsin Publishers; 1996.

58. Patterson JM. Families experiencing stress. Fam Syst Med 1988;6:202–37.

59. Willoughby BLB, Doty ND, Malik NM. Parental reactions to their child's sexual orientation disclosure: a family stress perspective. Parenting 2008;8(1):70–91.

60. D'Augelli AR, Hershberger SL, Pilkington NW. Lesbian, gay, and bisexual youth and their families: disclosure of sexual orientation and its consequences. Am J Orthopsychiatry 1998;68(3):361–71 [discussion: 372–5].

61. Padilla YC, Crisp C, Rew DL. Parental acceptance and illegal drug use among gay, lesbian, and bisexual adolescents: results from a national survey. Soc Work 2014;55(3):265–75.

62. D'Augelli AR, Grossman AH, Starks MT. Parents' awareness of lesbian, gay, and bisexual youths' sexual orientation. J Marriage Fam 2005;67(2):474–82.

63. Merighi JR, Grimes MD. Coming out to families in a multicultural context. Fam Soc 2000;81(1):32.

64. Newman BS, Muzzonigro PG. The effects of traditional family values on the coming out process of gay male adolescents. Adolescence 1993;28(109):213–26.

65. Needham BL, Austin EL. Sexual orientation, parental support, and health during the transition to young adulthood. J Youth Adolesc 2010;39(10):1189–98.

66. Horn SS. Attitudes about sexual orientation. In: Patterson CJ, D'Augelli AR, editors. Handbook of psychology and sexual orientation. New York: Oxford University Press; 2013. p. 239–51.

67. Ryan C, Huebner D, Diaz RM, et al. Family rejection as a predictor of negative health outcomes in white and Latino lesbian, gay, and bisexual young adults. Pediatrics 2009;123(1):346–52.

68. Poteat VP, Mereish EH, DiGiovanni CD, et al. The effects of general and homophobic victimization on adolescents' psychosocial and educational concerns: the importance of intersecting identities and parent support. J Couns Psychol 2011;58(4):597–609.

69. Yadegarfard M, Meinhold-Bergmann ME, Ho R. Family rejection, social isolation, and loneliness as predictors of negative health outcomes (depression, suicidal ideation, and sexual risk behavior) among Thai male-to-female transgender adolescents. J LGBT Youth 2014;11(4):347–63.

70. Bregman HR, Malik NM, Page MJL, et al. Identity profiles in lesbian, gay, and bisexual youth: the role of family influences. J Youth Adolesc 2013;42(3):417–30.

71. D'Augelli AR, Grossman AH, Starks MT, et al. Factors associated with parents' knowledge of gay, lesbian, and bisexual youths' sexual orientation. J GLBT Fam Stud 2010;6(2):178–98.

72. Ryan C, Russell ST, Huebner D, et al. Family acceptance in adolescence and the health of LGBT young adults. J Child Adolesc Psychiatr Nurs 2010;23(4):205–13.

73. Newcomb ME, Heinz AJ, Birkett M, et al. A longitudinal examination of risk and protective factors for cigarette smoking among lesbian, gay, bisexual and transgender youth. J Adolesc Health 2014;54(5):558–64.

74. Newcomb ME, Heinz AJ, Mustanski B. Examining risk and protective factors for alcohol use in lesbian, gay, bisexual, and transgender youth: a longitudinal multi-level analysis. J Stud Alcohol Drugs 2012;73(5):783–93. Available at: http://www.pubmedcentral.nih.gov/articlerender.fcgi?artid=3410946&tool=pmcentrez&rendertype=abstract.
75. Simons L, Schrager SM, Clark LF, Belzer M, Olson J. Parental support and mental health among transgender adolescents. J Adolesc Health 2013;53(6):791–3.

Human Immunodeficiency Virus, Other Sexually Transmitted Infections, and Sexual and Reproductive Health in Lesbian, Gay, Bisexual, Transgender Youth

 CrossMark

Sarah M. Wood, MD[a,b,*], Caroline Salas-Humara, MD[b], Nadia L. Dowshen, MD[c,d]

KEYWORDS

- STI • Sexual health • HIV • LGBT • Sexual minority • Gender minority
- Gender nonconforming • Adolescent

KEY POINTS

- Although lesbian, gay, bisexual, transgender (LGBT) youth face many sexual health inequities, including increased risk of human immunodeficiency virus (HIV), sexually transmitted infections (STIs), and pregnancy, providers have the opportunity to help young people to grow up to become sexually healthy adults.
- Pediatricians can support the development of healthy sexual identities and behavior by discussing sexual orientation and behavior in a nonjudgmental, respectful, and confidential manner.
- It is imperative to screen for HIV and recognize symptoms of acute HIV infection among all adolescents, but special attention should be paid to young men who have sex with men and young transgender women who are disproportionately affected; early diagnosis, linkage to, and retention in care with effective treatment improves both patient-specific and public health outcomes.

Continued

Disclosure Statement: The authors have nothing to disclose.
[a] Craig-Dalsimer Division of Adolescent Medicine, Children's Hospital of Philadelphia, 34th and Civic Center Boulevard, 11 Northwest Tower, Philadelphia, PA 19104, USA; [b] NYU Langone Fink Ambulatory Care Center, 160 East 32nd Street, 3rd Floor, New York, NY 10016, USA; [c] Department of Pediatrics, University of Pennsylvania School of Medicine, 34th and Civic Center Blvd, 9NW Tower, Philadelphia, PA, USA; [d] Craig-Dalsimer Division of Adolescent Medicine, Children's Hospital of Philadelphia, 34th and Civic Center Boulevard, 11 Northwest Tower, Philadelphia, PA 19104, USA
* Corresponding author. Craig-Dalsimer Division of Adolescent Medicine, Children's Hospital of Philadelphia, 34th and Civic Center Boulevard, 11 Northwest Tower, Philadelphia, PA 19104.
E-mail address: woodsa@email.chop.edu

Pediatr Clin N Am 63 (2016) 1027–1055
http://dx.doi.org/10.1016/j.pcl.2016.07.006
0031-3955/16/© 2016 Elsevier Inc. All rights reserved.
pediatric.theclinics.com

Continued

- LGBT youth, like their heterosexual counterparts, are at risk for syphilis, gonorrhea, chlamydia, trichomonas, and human papilloma virus (HPV), and providers should be familiar with the recommendations for screening of these STIs.
- Providers should offer sexual health preventive services, including safer sex counseling, HIV pre-exposure and postexposure prophylaxis, and vaccination for hepatitis A, B, and HPV, as well as discussion of sexual transmission of hepatitis C by HIV-infected men who have sex with men.

INTRODUCTION

Given estimates that more than 5% of the population identifies as lesbian, gay, bisexual, transgender (LGBT), or questioning, pediatricians are likely to care for LGBT youth at some point during practice. As health care providers, pediatricians are uniquely positioned to serve as expert guides to adolescents and young adults (AYA) navigating their sexuality and sexual health. By providing support and accurate information, pediatricians can positively influence those youth struggling with their sexuality, particularly those who are LGBT. It is important to understand that although this population may face unique challenges, pediatric providers can help ensure that they grow up to have healthy sexual and reproductive lives.

SEXUAL HEALTH AND REPRODUCTIVE HEALTH INEQUITIES AMONG LESBIAN, GAY, BISEXUAL, AND TRANSGENDER YOUTH
Epidemiology

Data demonstrate that LGBT youth are more likely than their heterosexual counterparts to experience a wide array of health inequities, many of which predispose them to an increased risk of sexually transmitted infections (STIs) and human immunodeficiency virus (HIV).[1] They are often subject to stigmatization, isolation, and societal and parental rejection. It is likely that these health inequities arise from individual, interpersonal, and structural stigma, which promote barriers to care (see Mark L. Hatzenbuehler and John E. Pachankis' article, "Stigma and Minority Stress as Social Determinants of Health Among LGBT Youth: Research Evidence and Clinical Implications," in this issue).[2]

LGBT youth also face significantly different sexual health outcomes related to sexual assault, STIs, HIV, and teen pregnancy. They are at significantly higher risk of sexual assault and abuse than their heterosexual peers.[3] In addition, according to Youth Risk Behavioral Surveillance data, compared with heterosexual youth, LGBT youth are more likely to be sexually active, to have earlier sexual debut (before age 13), and have 4 or more sexual partners.[4] Compared with heterosexual youth, LGBT youth were about half as likely to have used a condom at last intercourse (35.8% vs 65.5%). These behaviors may partly explain why although the overall incidence rates of gonorrhea, chlamydia, and syphilis have decreased among adolescents in the last 15 years, they have increased among adolescent men who have sex with men (MSM).[5] Adolescent MSM have also been disproportionately affected by HIV. Although MSM accounted for only 4% of the male population in the United States in 2010,[6] they represented 78% of new HIV infections among men and 68% of total new infections. Over the past decade, HIV incidence in young MSM of color has increased by 87%.[7] Young transgender women (YTW) are particularly vulnerable to HIV. A review of studies estimated that HIV prevalence for transgender women was nearly 50 times as high as that of other adults.[8]

Although providers need to be aware of the epidemiology of STIs in LGBT youth, they should use caution in making assumptions about their patient's sexual practices. It is important to remember that the high STI rates in LGBT youth are not necessarily due to an increased number of partners or frequency of sex. For MSM, the anatomy and immunology of the rectal mucosa lead to a higher biologic susceptibility to STIs and HIV. Racial disparities also play a role in the increased incidence of HIV in young men and transgender women of color who have sex with men. Although rates of unprotected anal intercourse are similar between African American and other MSM, African American MSM are more likely to experience structural barriers such as unemployment, lack of health insurance, incarceration, or lower educational attainment levels that may act as barriers to care and thus increase the risk of HIV.[9] Similarly, it is important to remember that for LGBT youth, sexual behavior does not necessarily align with reported sexual attraction and identity, which are other aspects of sexual orientation that may change over time. For example, many women who have sex with women (WSW) have current or past male partners, and data show they may be less likely to use effective contraception and are at increased risk for pregnancy.[10]

Health care providers, equipped with knowledge and expertise, have the opportunity to mitigate these sexual health inequities with each valuable patient encounter. Please see Scott E. Hadland and colleagues' article, "Caring for LGBT Youth and Families in Inclusive and Affirmative Environments," in this issue, for review of appropriate terminology used to describe gender identity and sexual orientation.

APPROACH TO SEXUAL AND REPRODUCTIVE HEALTH CARE FOR LESBIAN, GAY, BISEXUAL, TRANSGENDER YOUTH

It is the health care provider's responsibility to openly discuss matters of sexual health, including sexual orientation, sexual behavior, and gender identity, with patients. If they do not, they risk losing valuable opportunities both to provide a safe and accepting setting for youth to voice concerns and questions and to intervene for those youth in crisis. It is also important to recognize that some LGBT youth may be reluctant to openly discuss matters of sexual health and sexuality without first establishing a trusting relationship with their provider. It may take repeated visits before addressing sexual health in detail. The urgency of this discussion will, in part, be directed by the patient's complaint; if a patient presents for suspected STI, then discussion regarding sexual risk may be accelerated. Providers must keep in mind that it is not the role of the clinician to identify LGBT youth, but rather simply provide an open, accepting setting if they wish to discuss sexual health.

Discussing Sexual Health and Sexuality

Confidentiality

Every effort should be made to maintain confidentiality with the patient at all levels of care from front desk staff to parental access to protected information. Clinicians should familiarize themselves with their region's laws and statutes regarding a minor's access to confidential sexual health services and be prepared to discuss these with patients and parents. Detailed information regarding individual state policies can be found at the Guttmacher Institute[11] (http://www.guttmacher.org/statecenter/spibs/spib_MASS.pdf).

It is essential that clinicians meet with their adolescent patients without a parent present to best allow for open communication. When discussing confidentiality with a patient, it may be helpful to use the word "private" instead of "confidential," because teens may misinterpret the word confidential to denote "confidence."[12] For example, you might say: "I am using the word 'confidential,' which is another way of saying 'private,' and what this means is that I will do my best not to spread your business around to your parents or anyone else." During this conversation with the young person, in order to maintain trust, it is also important to be explicit about the limits of privacy. As mentioned above, this includes being familiar with your region's laws regarding privacy so that you can communicate them clearly. Generally, professional ethics, law, and regulation may limit nonemancipated or nonmature minors' privilege of confidentiality and require clinically appropriate reporting to ensure safety when a patient is in imminent danger (for example, in cases of child abuse, suicidal or homicidal intent, or life-threatening substance abuse). These exceptions are distinct from areas in which confidentiality may be protected by ethics and locally applicable law and regulation, such as matters of consensual sex, contraception, diagnosis and treatment of STIs, and other matters of sexual and reproductive health.[12] When uncertain, clinicians should consider seeking child protective, ethical, and/or legal consultation to help guide them.

Setting the stage for nonjudgment, respect, and honesty

Providers can set the tone of comfort by outlining 3 basic tenets of care with the patient: a nonjudgmental approach, respect, and honesty.[12] Patients should understand your role: to guide and help them to transition into being self-advocates. Many LGBT youth may expect to be judged given their past experiences with other health care providers and authority figures. It is helpful to remind them that you will serve them in a nonjudgmental way. You may ask patients what they prefer to be called with the parents in the room, and again when they are alone. Last, youth should understand that you will provide them with honest and accurate information.

Taking a sexual history

When taking a sexual history, use language that is inclusive and ask questions that are open-ended and nonjudgmental. For example, use gender-neutral language when inquiring about potential partners. In addition, providers should remember sexuality is a multidimensional and fluid construct, which may evolve throughout the course of adolescence. Sexual identity and sexual behavior are not synonymous, and providers should take caution not to make assumptions that identity predicts behavior. Providers can use the Attraction, Behavior, Orientation framework as a guide in sexual history taking (**Box 1**). Consider asking youth if they have questions about any sexual behaviors, regardless of whether they have experienced them. When tailoring questions to youth regarding sexual experiences, remember that sexual orientation or attraction does not predict sexual behavior. WSW can engage in sexual behavior leading to pregnancy, so should be asked about their need for contraception. HIV testing for MSM should be approached in the same manner as it would for any at-risk adolescent and should not be the sole focus of care. Remember that sexual practices may not be dissimilar for heterosexual, gay, lesbian, and bisexual youth.[13] For example, although a youth may identify as heterosexual, it does not necessarily mean that he or she does not engage in anal sex. In fact, 44% of heterosexual men and 36% of heterosexual women admitted to having had anal sex at least once in their lives according to a recent report.[14]

It is important to do a complete review of symptoms, asking concretely about symptoms of STIs. Youth may not offer these symptoms unless expressly asked about them. Providers should ask about vaginal or penile discharge, abdominal or back pain, dysuria, vomiting, dyspareunia, after-coital bleeding, genital lesions, and anorectal symptoms consistent with proctitis such as rectal discharge or bleeding, tenesmus, or pain during anal intercourse. Ask about menstrual and STI histories, as well as

---

Box 1
Sexual history questions using the attraction, behavior, orientation framework

Sexual attraction

- Have you ever had a crush or been romantically involved with a boy or girl? Do you know if you are sexually attracted to men, women, or both?
- Are you dating someone? If so, tell me about this person and what that relationship is like.

Sexual behavior

- Have you ever done anything sexually, like kissing, or touching in areas below the waist with a girl or boy?
- Do you have sex with men (boys), women (girls), or both?
- Do you or have you had vaginal sex? Oral sex? Anal sex?
- For anal sex: does your partner put his penis in your anus or vice versa or both?
- How many partners have you had in the last 6 months?
- How do you protect yourself against sexually transmitted diseases and pregnancy?
- Do you use condoms for anal or vaginal sex? If so, how many times out of 10 do you use them?
- Do you have sex with anyone other than your boyfriend or girlfriend? If so, how often are you using condoms?
- Has anyone ever forced you to do something sexually that you did not wish to do?
- Have you ever needed to trade sex for money, drugs, or a safe place to stay?
- Have you ever been diagnosed with gonorrhea, chlamydia, syphilis, herpes, HIV, or another STI?
- Do you use recreational drugs when you have sex? Crystal meth? Alcohol? Cocaine? Others?

Sexual orientation and disclosure

- How would you describe your sexual orientation? For example, do you consider yourself gay, straight, lesbian, bisexual, or queer, or are you not sure or do not wish to label it?
- Have you ever talked to anyone in your family or your friends or any other adult besides me about "coming out"? How did they react?
- It is normal for people to sometimes be confused about their sexual feelings and experiences. Do you have any questions you would like to ask me about this?

Data from Dowshen N, Hawkins L, Arrington-Sanders R, et al. Sexual and gender minority youth. In: Ginsberg K, editor. Reaching teens: strength based communication strategies to build resilience and support healthy adolescent development. Elk Grove (IL): AAP Press; 2014. p. 531–8.

---

history of forced or coercive sex. Providers should ask about any new partners in the last 3 months as a gauge of whether patients need more frequent STI testing.

Physical Examination

When approaching the physical examination with LGBT youth, consider whether it is necessary to perform the genital examination on first encounter. It may be helpful to establish a therapeutic alliance with a patient over subsequent encounters. Although no data exist on the percentage of trans youth who have undergone gender affirmation surgery, it is likely that most transmen and transwomen, particularly youth, have not undergone gender affirmation surgery, especially given that the official standard of the 2 organizations that provide standards of care for transgender individuals

(World Professional Association for Transgender Health and the Endocrine Society) recommend to defer genital surgery until the transitioning individual has reached 18 years of age. Most transgender patients, therefore, still have their natal sexual organs, which can be a great source of dysphoria and discomfort for the patient. Therefore, when performing genital examinations in these patients, the clinician should be aware that this experience may be particularly stressful because they may not identify with their anatomy (ie, examining the testicles of a transgender person who was born a boy, but identifies as a woman). Always prepare the patient by describing exactly what you are going to do and why you are doing it. Place patients in control by letting them know that you will discontinue the examination at any point if they wish. For transgender patients, physical examination for cancer screening should be dictated by the anatomy of the patient, and not gender identity. Routine testicular examinations should be performed for transgender women who have not had their testicles removed. Cervical cancer screening should be performed for transgender men according to guidelines. Anal STI screening should be performed for those youth who have anal intercourse regardless of sex, sexual orientation, or gender identity.

SEXUALLY TRANSMITTED INFECTIONS IN LESBIAN, GAY, BISEXUAL, TRANSGENDER YOUTH

Among LGBT youth, clinicians should be vigilant about screening for STIs to decrease patient morbidity, prevent secondary STI transmission, and to decrease the risk of HIV acquisition.

STIs, particularly genital ulcerative disease, serve as key risk factors for HIV infection in AYA. Genital ulcer disease in HIV-infected individuals can increase the risk of transmission due to increase in HIV viral shedding; conversely, in HIV-uninfected individuals, disruption of the mucosal barrier and increased number of antigen-presenting cells increase the risk of HIV acquisition.[15–17] Clinicians should at minimum follow existing guidelines for STI and HIV screening for LGBT youth and increase frequency of screening in the setting of symptoms or high-risk behavior.

Human Immunodeficiency Virus in Adolescents

Although the overall incidence of HIV infection in the United States has plateaued in recent years, the rates of new infection are increasing among AYA, particularly among young MSM of color. Despite ongoing HIV prevention outreach and education efforts, AYA aged 13 to 29 accounted for 26% of all new infections in the United States in 2010.[18] Specifically, young black MSM are facing the steepest increases in new infection; the rates of new infection in this population increased by 87% in the last decade (Fig. 1). Compared with adults, young MSM are less likely to be aware of their positive HIV status (~49% vs 80% of adults), initiate HIV care, start antiretroviral therapy (ART), or achieve a suppressed viral load, which leads to increased morbidity among youth living with HIV.[19]

Early identification of infection and initiation of treatment can lead to health benefits on the public and individual level. In particular, clinicians should maintain a high index of suspicion for acute HIV infection (AHI) when evaluating adolescents with nonspecific febrile illnesses or mononucleosis-like syndrome as well as in adolescents with a recent high-risk exposure or STI. An estimated 50% to 89% of patients with AHI are symptomatic and most commonly present with fever, lymphadenopathy, pharyngitis, rash, myalgias, mucocutaneous ulcers, or headache.[20,21] Clinicians should be familiar with the appropriate HIV tests to capture AHI (Table 1).

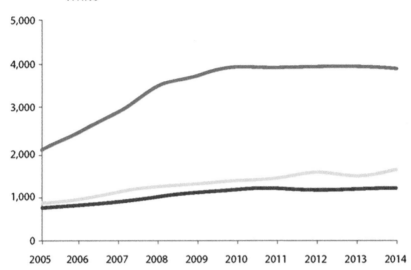

Fig. 1. HIV diagnoses among MSM age 13 to 24 by race and ethnicity, 2005 to 2014. (*From* Centers for Disease Control and Prevention. CDC Fact Sheet: Trends in U.S. HIV Diagnoses, 2005–2014 February. 2016.)

Table 1
Screening, diagnosis, and treatment of human immunodeficiency virus infection

	Screening & Diagnosis of HIV		
Specimen Source	**Test**	**Time to Positivity (d)**	**Screening Frequency**
Blood	HIV Ag/Ab test[a]	~15–30	• At least annually if sexually active
Blood/oral fluid	HIV rapid immunoassay[b]	~22–35	• All who seek treatment or evaluation for STIs
			• All 13–64 y (opt-out)[c]
Blood	HIV RNA Qualitative or Quantitative assay	~10	If symptoms of AHI

Treatment
ART is now recommended for all adolescents and adults living with HIV, irrespective of CD4$^+$ cell count or viral load, to reduce the risk of disease progression and secondary transmission of HIV.

[a] Fourth-generation assay detects HIV-1 and -2-specific antibodies and p24-specific antigen.
[b] Third-generation immunoassay detecting HIV-specific immunoglobulin M.
[c] CDC recommends screening at 13 to 64 y; the USPSTF recommends screening from 15 to 65 y.
Data from Workowski KA, Bolan GA, Centers for Disease Control and Prevention. Sexually transmitted diseases treatment guidelines, 2015. MMWR Recomm Rep 2015;64(RR-03):1–137; and Panel on Antiretroviral Guidelines for Adults and Adolescents. Guidelines for the use of antiretroviral agents in HIV-1-infected adults and adolescents. Department of Health and Human Services. Available at http://aidsinfo.nih.gov/contentfiles/lvguidelines/AdultandAdolescentGL.pdf.

Human immunodeficiency virus testing

Because of the numerous individual and public health benefits of early recognition and treatment of HIV, the Centers for Disease Control and Prevention (CDC), American Academy of Pediatrics (AAP), and US Preventative Services Task Force (USPSTF) all recommend routine screening of sexually active adolescents (see **Table 1**). The AAP also encourages testing of all youth by the age of 16 to 18 regardless of sexual report, because many youth may underreport sexual activity.[22] In 2014, the CDC updated their recommendations regarding laboratory testing for HIV infection,[23] recommending initial testing with a US Food and Drug Administration (FDA)-approved antigen/antibody combination (fourth-generation) assay that detects both HIV-1 and HIV-2 antibody as well as HIV-1 p24 antigen. This assay has increased sensitivity in detecting early HIV infection, because the p24 antigen is expressed during acute infection when antibodies are not yet detectable. Positive fourth-generation assays should be confirmed by an immunoassay for HIV-specific antibodies. Rapid blood or oral fluid–based antibody-based tests have the advantage of results delivery at the point of care. However, these third-generation assays may miss those patients in acute infection. For patients with substantial concern for AHI, a nucleic acid amplification test (NAAT) in the form of a quantitative or qualitative HIV RNA assay has the highest sensitivity for diagnosing patients within the "window" period.

Delivering results and linkage to care

Delivering negative HIV results is an opportunity for counseling regarding STIs and HIV infection, and connection to prevention services, such as HIV pre-exposure prophylaxis (PrEP). Positive results should be discussed with the patient in person and not over the telephone. It is important to convey a message of hope, while not diminishing the sadness and fear that may accompany the diagnosis. With early initiation of ART, AYA with HIV can be expected to lead long, healthy, and productive lives. Providers should assess for patient safety and establish a plan for close follow-up. Every effort should be made to immediately link the patient to a care team with adolescent HIV expertise so that ART can be started. Recent data from the START trial has demonstrated that immediate initiation of ART, irrespective of $CD4^+$ cell counts and viral loads, can reduce the risk of serious AIDS-related events (such as AIDS-related cancer), serious nonrelated AIDS events (such as cardiovascular, renal, and liver disease), and overall mortality compared with patients in which ART was deferred.[24] In addition, initiation of treatment during AHI may reduce the size of the latent viral reservoir.[25] Providers should be aware of resources for treatment in their area and can contact local health departments to facilitate linkage to care.

Chlamydial Infections

Chlamydia is the most common reported bacterial STI in the United States and is highly prevalent among young women and MSM. Rectal and pharyngeal chlamydia prevalence rates among screened MSM have been reported to be 3% to 10.5%[26] and 0.5% to 2.3%,[27] respectively. WSW are at substantial risk for chlamydia infection as well; one study estimated that *Chlamydia trachomatis* infection was higher in women reporting same sex sexual behavior.[28] Because screening programs have been shown to reduce rates of pelvic inflammatory disease (PID), the CDC recommends routine annual screening for all sexually active women less than 25 years of age.[29] Because of their high risk of infection, the CDC also recommends that MSM be screened at least annually for urethral infection as well as rectal infection in men who have had receptive anal intercourse (**Table 2**).

Table 2
Screening, diagnosis, and treatment of chlamydial infections

		Screening & Diagnosis		
Specimen		**Screening Frequency**		
Source	**Test**	**MSM**	**Females**	**Persons with HIV**
Urine	NAAT	• At least annually if sexually active • Every 3–6 mo if at increased risk • If symptomatic		For sexually active persons, screen at initial evaluation and then at least annually thereafter
Cervix/vagina	NAAT	—	• Yearly if sexually active • If symptomatic	For sexually active persons, screen at initial evaluation and then at least annually thereafter
Throat	NAAT or culture[a]	Not recommended		
Anus	NAAT or culture[a]	• At least annually if sexually active • Every 3–6 mo if increased risk or symptomatic	If report receptive anal sex or if symptomatic	For sexually active persons, screen at initial evaluation and then at least annually thereafter

	Treatment	
Site of Infection	**Recommended Regimen**	**Alternative Regimens**
Uncomplicated genital/rectal/pharyngeal infections	• Azithromycin 1 g po in a single dose or • Doxycycline 100 mg po bid × 7 d	• Erythromycin base 500 mg po qid × 7 d or • Erythromycin ethylsuccinate 800 mg po qid × 7 d or • Levofloxacin 500 mg po qd × 7 d or • Ofloxacin 300 mg po bid × 7 d
Pregnant women[b]	Azithromycin 1 g po in a single dose	• Amoxicillin 500 mg po tid × 7 d • Erythromycin base 500 mg po qid × 7 d or • Erythromycin base 250 mg po qid × 14 d or • Erythromycin ethylsuccinate 800 mg po qid × 7 d or • Erythromycin ethylsuccinate 400 mg po qid ×14 d
Lymphogranuloma venereum	Doxycycline 100 mg po bid × 21 d	Erythromycin base 500 mg po qid × 21 d

[a] Although NAAT has superior sensitivity and specificity to culture in diagnosing rectal GC and chlamydia, not all laboratory tests are Clinical Laboratory Improvement Amendment (CLIA) certified for oropharyngeal and rectal specimens.
[b] Every effort to use a recommended regimen should be made. Test-of-cure follow-up (preferably by NAAT) 3 to 4 weeks after completion of therapy is recommended in pregnancy.
    Data from Workowski KA, Bolan GA, Centers for Disease Control and Prevention. Sexually transmitted diseases treatment guidelines, 2015. MMWR Recomm Rep 2015;64(RR-03):1–137.

Chlamydial infection in men having sex with men

Although there are many manifestations of chlamydia, it is important to remember that most infections are asymptomatic. *C trachomatis* is the most common cause of non-gonoccocal urethritis in men, typically presenting with watery, scant urethral discharge and dysuria. Epididymitis is typically characterized by unilateral testicular pain, swelling, and tenderness. Chlamydial proctitis occurs primarily in MSM who engage in receptive anal intercourse. Symptoms typically include diarrhea, rectal pain or bleeding, tenesmus, and rectal discharge. However, rectal chlamydia is commonly asymptomatic. When evaluating MSM with rectal symptoms, it is important to also consider lymphogranuloma venereum (caused by *C trachomatis* serovars L1-L3), which may cause a proctocolitis, often mimicking inflammatory bowel disease. It is imperative to recognize proctitis because it is associated with an up to 9-fold risk of HIV acquisition,[30] and a diagnosis of proctitis in MSM warrants evaluation for HIV and other STIs. Patients should be treated empirically while awaiting diagnostic results (**Table 3**).

Chlamydial infection in women having sex with women

Chlamydial infection in WSW presents in the same manner as in their heterosexual counterparts, namely with cervicitis, urethritis, PID, and perihepatitis (Fitz-Hugh-Curtis syndrome). Any young woman with symptoms of cervicitis accompanied by abdominal pain, fever, back pain, or dyspareunia should have a pelvic examination to assess for PID. Early treatment reduces the risk for complications, including infertility, tubo-ovarian abscess, and chronic pelvic pain (see **Table 3**).

Gonococcal Infections

Neisseria gonorrhea is the second most common bacterial STI. Prevalence rates of gonorrhea among MSM at STI clinics are estimated to be 15.3% with even higher rates in HIV-infected patients.[31] Rates of gonorrhea transmission in WSW are largely unknown, and risk likely varies depending on the sexual practice with digital-vaginal, digital-anal, and/or penetrative toys presenting a route for infection via cervical secretions[32] (**Table 4**).

Gonococcal infection in men having sex with men

Gonococcal (GC) urethritis in men most commonly presents with urethral discharge that is purulent and copious. GC may also cause epididymitis; however, most infections are caused by *C trachomatis*. Most cases of anorectal GC in both men and women are asymptomatic, but may present with the same symptoms of chlamydial proctitis detailed above. GC proctitis is indistinguishable from other organisms that cause proctitis, and like chlamydial infection, also incurs an increased risk of HIV acquisition.[30]

Gonococcal infection in women having sex with women

Similar to infection with *C trachomatis*, infection in women can lead to urethritis, cervicitis, or PID.

Gonococcal infections of the pharynx

Pharyngeal gonorrhea is more efficiently spread by oral-penile than oral-vaginal contact. Most infections are asymptomatic. When symptoms are present, sore throat, pharyngeal exudate, and/or cervical lymphadenitis are common. Although the bacterial concentrations are lower in the pharynx, it is thought to be a reservoir for drug-resistant types.[33] GC infections of the pharynx are more difficult to eradicate than urogenital and anorectal infections. Because the CDC's Gonococcal Isolate

Table 3
Empiric treatment of pelvic inflammatory disease and bacterial sexually transmitted infections

	Treatment	
Site of Infection	**Recommended Regimen**	**Alternative Regimens**

PID: Outpatient treatment	• Ceftriaxone 250 mg intramuscularly (IM) in a single dose
	  OR
	• Cefoxitin 2 g IM AND Probenecid 1 g po in a single dose
	  OR
	• Other parental third-generation cephalosporin
	  PLUS
	• Doxycycline 100 mg po bid × 14 d[a]
	• ±Metronidazole 500 mg po bid × 5 d	

PID: Parenteral treatment[b]	• Either Cefotetan 2 g IV every 12 h
	  OR
	• Cefoxitin 2 g IV every 6 h
	  PLUS
	• Doxycycline 100 mg po or IV every 12 h[a]
	  OR
	• Clindamycin 900 mg IV q 8 h
	  PLUS
	• Gentamicin 2 mg/kg IV or IM loading dose followed by 1.5 mg/kg every 8 h[c]
		• Ampicillin/Sulbactam 3 g IV q 6 h
		  PLUS
		• Doxycycline 100 mg po or IV q 12 h

Cervicitis	• Azithromycin 1 g po in a single dose OR • Doxycycline 100 mg po bid × 7 d[a]	

Nongonococcal urethritis	• Azithromycin 1 g po in a single dose
	  OR
	• Doxycycline 100 mg po bid × 7 d[a]
		• Erythromycin base 500 mg po qid × 7 d
		  OR
		• Erythromycin ethylsuccinate 800 mg po qid × 7 d
		  OR
		• Levofloxacin 500 mg po qd × 7 d
		  OR
		• Ofloxacin 300 mg po bid × 7 d

Epididymitis	Likely due to gonorrhea or chlamydia
	• Ceftriaxone 250 mg IM in a single dose
	  PLUS
	• Doxycycline 100 mg bid × 10 d
	Likely due to enteric organisms (men who practice insertive anal sex)[d]
	• Ceftriaxone 250 mg IM in a single dose
	  PLUS
	• Levofloxacin 500 mg po daily × 10 d[c]
	  OR
	• Ofloxacin 300 mg po bid × 10 d[c]	

(continued on next page)

Table 3 (continued)		
Treatment		
Site of Infection	**Recommended Regimen**	**Alternative Regimens**
Proctitis	• Ceftriaxone 250 mg IM in a single dose PLUS • Doxycycline 100 mg bid × 7 d[a]	

[a] Contraindicated for pregnant and nursing women.
[b] Discontinue IV therapy 24 h after patient improves clinically and continue with oral therapy for a total of 14 d.
[c] May use gentamicin single daily dosing of 3-5 mg/kg.
[d] If gonorrhea is documented, change to a medication regimen that does not include a fluoroquinolone.
Data from Workowski KA, Bolan GA, Centers for Disease Control and Prevention. Sexually transmitted diseases treatment guidelines. MMWR Recomm Rep 2015;64(RR-03):1–137.

Surveillance Project has documented rising rates of cefixime-resistant *N gonorrhoeae*, oral cephalosporins are no longer recommended for the treatment of any type of GC infection, including those of the pharynx[15] (see **Table 4**).

Disseminated gonococcal infection
Last, DGI presents in 0.5% to 3% of patients and manifests as 2 distinct clinical syndromes: purulent arthritis or a triad of tenosynovitis, dermatitis (petechial or pustular acral lesions), and polyarthralgias. Prompt recognition of DGI is critical, because it requires prolonged parenteral treatment and can lead to joint destruction if untreated.

Bacterial Vaginosis

Bacterial vaginosis (BV) is the most common cause of vaginal discharge in women of reproductive age.[34] BV results from replacement of the normal *Lactobacillus* species in the vagina with high concentrations of anaerobic organisms, typically resulting in copious, malodorous discharge and vaginal irritation. Although sexual transmission of BV has not been established, sexual activity is a known risk factor for BV.[35]

Although there are few studies in WSW, BV appears to be highly prevalent (25%–50%) in this population[36,37] and is associated with an increased number of female sexual partners, a female partner with BV symptoms, and receptive oral sex.[36,38,39] One randomized controlled trial in WSW demonstrated that reducing transmission of vaginal fluid through gloves and condom use for sex toys did not reduce recurrence[40]; however, further research needs to be conducted to elucidate sexual transmission via WSW. BV is associated with an increased risk of HIV, STIs, and pregnancy complications, and prompt treatment is therefore indicated (**Table 5**).

Trichomonal Infections

Trichomonas vaginalis (TV), a flagellated protozoa, is the most common nonviral STI worldwide. Most infected persons have minimal or no symptoms, and untreated infection can last for months to years. Women typically present with malodorous, yellow-green vaginal discharge with or without vulvar irritation. In men, symptoms consist of urethritis, epididymitis, or prostatitis. It is unclear if anal receptive sex may serve as mode of transmission and a reservoir for TV, because the prevalence of trichomoniasis in MSM is low.[41] However, male partners of women diagnosed with trichonomal infections should be treated, and treatment should be considered in men with persistent or treatment-resistant urethritis (**Table 6**). Trichomonal infection is associated with

Table 4
Screening, diagnosis, and treatment of gonococcal infections

Screening & Diagnosis

Specimen Source	Test	Screening Frequency		Persons with HIV
		Male	**Female**	
Urine	NAAT	• At least annually if sexually active, regardless of condom use • Every 3–6 mo if at increased risk • If symptomatic	• Yearly if sexually active • If symptomatic	For sexually active persons, screen at initial evaluation and then at least annually thereafter
Vaginal[a]	NAAT	—		
Throat		• At least annually if sexually active, regardless of condom use • Every 3–6 mo if at increased risk • If symptomatic	If report receptive oral sex and symptomatic	
Anus	NAAT or Culture[b]	• At least annually if sexually active, regardless of condom use • Every 3–6 mo if at increased risk • If symptomatic	If report receptive anal sex and symptomatic	

Treatment

Site of Infection	Recommended Regimen	Alternative Regimens
Uncomplicated genital/rectal infections	• Ceftriaxone 250 mg IM in a single dose PLUS • Azithromycin 1 g po in a single dose	• Cefixime 400 mg in a single dose[c] PLUS • Azithromycin 1 g po in a single dose If allergic to cephalosporins or severe penicillin allergy • Gemifloxicin 320 mg po or Gentamicin 240 mg IM PLUS • Azithromycin 2 g po in a single dose
Pharyngeal infections	• Ceftriaxone 250 mg IM in a single dose PLUS • Azithromycin 1 g po in a single dose	
Arthritis and arthritis-dermatitis syndrome	• Ceftriaxone 1g IM or IV every 24 h PLUS • Azithromycin 1 g po in a single dose	• Cefotaxime 1 g IV every 8 h OR • Cefitzoxime 1 g IV every 8 h PLUS • Azithromycin 1 g po
Gonoccocal meningitis and endocarditis	• Ceftriaxone 1-2 g IV every 12–24 h PLUS • Azithromycin 1 g po in a single dose	

[a] Although vaginal swabs are preferred over urine swabs for women, the sensitivity of urine NAAT approaches that of vaginal, and ease of specimen collection makes urine testing far more feasible in clinical practice.
[b] Not all laboratories are CLIA certified for oropharyngeal and rectal specimens, although NAAT has superior sensitivity and specificity in diagnosing rectal GC and chlamydia. Clinicians should be aware of their laboratory ability to assess pharyngeal NAAT.
[c] Only if ceftriaxone is unavailable.

Data from Workowski KA, Bolan GA, Centers for Disease Control and Prevention. Sexually transmitted diseases treatment guidelines, 2015. MMWR Recomm Rep 2015;64(RR-03):1–137.

Table 5
Screening, diagnosis, and treatment of bacterial vaginosis

	Screening & Diagnosis	
Specimen Source	**Test**	**Screening Frequency**
Vaginal fluid	• Microscopy w/wet mount OR • Amstel's clinical criteria (need 3 of 4): (1) homogenous, thin white discharge, (2) >50% clue cells on microscopy, (3) vaginal fluid pH >4.5, (4) fishy odor of vaginal fluid before or after addition of potassium hydroxide (whiff test)	Asymptomatic screening not recommended Test symptomatic female patients

	Treatment	
Site of Infection	**Recommended Regimen**	**Alternative Regimens**
Vaginal[c]	• Metronidazole 500 mg po bid × 7 d OR • Metronidazole gel 0.75%, 1 applicator (5 g) intravaginally, once daily × 5 d OR • Clindamycin cream 2%, 1 applicator (5 g) intravaginally, once daily × 7 d[b]	• Tinidazole[a] 2 g po daily × 2 d OR • Tinidazole 1 g po daily × 5 d OR • Clindamycin 300 mg po bid × 7 d OR • Clindamycin ovules 100 mg intravaginally at bedtime × 3 d

[a] Safety in pregnancy has not been established; pregnancy category C.
[b] May weaken latex condoms and contraceptive diaphragms.
[c] Treatment of male partners has not been shown to prevent recurrence in women.
  Data from Workowski KA, Bolan GA, Centers for Disease Control and Prevention. Sexually transmitted diseases treatment guidelines, 2015. MMWR Recomm Rep 2015;64(RR-03):1–137.

a 2- to 3-fold increased risk of HIV acquisition,[42] and among women with HIV, TV is associated with an increased risk for PID.[43]

Syphilis

Among YMSM, syphilis rates continue to increase, with 2013 having the highest incidence in cases among 15 to 19 year olds since 1995.[16] Syphilis, caused by the spirochete *Treponema pallidum*, may present in primary (typically a solitary painless called a chancre), secondary (disseminated findings such as maculopapular rash involving palms/soles, cutaneous lesions, and lymphadenopathy), or tertiary (cardiac, gummatous, or neurosensory impairment) stages. In addition, patients may present with central nervous system involvement (neurosyphilis), such as meningitis, cranial neuropathy, and altered mental status at any stage of the disease. Finally, asymptomatic patients may be diagnosed with latent syphilis, defined as seroreactivity without evidence of primary, secondary, or tertiary syphilis. Early latent syphilis is diagnosed in those who acquired syphilis in the year before diagnosis, as evidenced by a documented seroconversion or greater than 2 week, 4-fold or greater increase in treponemal titers, prior symptoms of primary or secondary syphilis, or a partner in the preceding year with documented syphilis. Late latent syphilis is diagnosed in asymptomatic patients if the above criteria are not met in the year before diagnosis.

Table 6
Screening, diagnosis, and treatment guidelines of trichomonal infections

		Screening & Diagnosis		
		Screening Frequency		
Specimen Source	Test	M	F	Persons with HIV
Vaginal (collected by patient or provider)	Wet mount with direct visualization of flagellated, motile, pear-shaped organisms on saline wet mount microscopy OR OSOM rapid test OR Affirm nucleic acid probe test	—	• Consider for women receiving care in high-prevalence settings (ie, STD clinics) and at high risk (ie, multiple sexual partners, history of STD) • If symptomatic	• For women at entry to care and at least annually thereafter • If symptomatic

	Treatment	
Site of Infection	Recommended Regimen	Alternative Regimens
All sites	• Metronidazole 2 g po in a single dose OR • Tinidazole 2 g po in a single dose[a]	Metronidazole 500 mg po bid × 7 d
Infection in HIV-positive women	• Metronidazole 500 mg bid × 7d	

[a] Safety in pregnancy has not been established; pregnancy category C.
Data from Workowski KA, Bolan GA, Centers for Disease Control and Prevention. Sexually transmitted diseases treatment guidelines, 2015. MMWR Recomm Rep 2015;64(RR-03):1–137.

Syphilis is diagnosed via 2-stage testing: a nontreponemal test (venereal disease research laboratory [VDRL] or rapid plasma reagin [RPR]), followed by a treponemal test (fluorescent treponemal antibody absorbed or passive particle agglutination). In early primary syphilis, RPR and VDRL may be negative, and definitive diagnosis requires darkfield microscopy of the lesion exudate. However, as this is often not available, patients with a chancre or a recent high-risk exposure should be treated empirically. Treatment course is dependent on clinical stage or length of latency (**Table 7**). Syphilis and HIV are known to be co-occurring, and a new syphilis diagnosis should prompt immediate testing for HIV.[15,16]

Hepatitis

Hepatitis A, B, and C may all take the form of STIs in youth. Hepatitis A viral (HAV) infection is a self-limited disease primarily transmitted via the fecal-oral route, and therefore, may arise from oral-anal sexual contact. Acute HAV typically presents with fever, jaundice, nausea, and gastrointestinal (GI) upset and is treated with supportive care. Hepatitis B virus (HBV) may be transmitted through blood, seminal fluid, or vaginal fluid and can lead to either an acute and self-limited illness or chronic infection. Routine immunization against HBV in infancy has resulted in a largely immune adolescent population in the United States. However, young adults who have not been immunized, teens whose immunity has waned, or youth who engage in MSM or injection drug use (IDU) behavior remain at risk. Although hepatitis C virus

Table 7
Screening, diagnosis, and treatment of syphilis

Screening & Diagnosis			
Specimen Source	**Test**	**Screening Frequency**		**Persons with HIV**
		Male	**Female**	
Blood	RPR or VDRL with reflex treponemal test	• At least annually if sexually active • Every 3–6 mo if increased risk	Not recommended	At first HIV evaluation and then at least annually thereafter

Treatment		
Stage of Disease	**Recommended Regimen**	**Alternative Regimens**[a]
Primary, secondary, and early latent syphilis	Benzathine penicillin G 2.4 million units in a single dose	• Doxycycline 100 mg po bid × 14 d OR • Tetracycline 500 mg po qid × 14 d OR • Ceftriaxone 1 g IM or IV qd × 10–14 d
Late latent and latent of unknown duration	Benzathine penicillin G 7.2 million units total, administered as 3 doses of 2.4 million units IM at 1-wk intervals	• Doxycycline 100 mg po bid × 28 d OR • Tetracycline 500 mg po qid × 28 d
Tertiary syphilis with normal CSF	Benzathine penicillin G 7.2 million units total, administered as 3 doses of 2.4 million units IM at 1-wk intervals	
Neurosyphilis and ocular syphilis[b]	Aqueous crystalline penicillin G 18–24 million units per day, administered as 3–4 million units IV every 4 h or continuous infusion for 10–14 d	• Procaine penicillin G, 2.4 million units IM qd × 10–14 d PLUS • Probenecid 500 mg po qid × 10–14 d

[a] Alternates should be used only for penicillin-allergic patients. Efficacy of these therapies has not been established. Compliance these regimens is difficult, and close follow-up is essential. If compliance or follow-up cannot be ensured, or if the patient is pregnant, the patient should be desensitized and treated with benzathine penicillin.
[b] Some specialists recommend 2.4 million units of benzathine penicillin G every week for up to 3 wk after completion of neurosyphilis treatment.
Data from Workowski KA, Bolan GA, Centers for Disease Control and Prevention. Sexually transmitted diseases treatment guidelines, 2015. MMWR Recomm Rep 2015;64(RR-03):1–137.

(HCV) is the most common blood-borne infection in the United States, sexual transmission of HCV is uncommon among AYA. The exception to this is among MSM, particularly those with HIV, who represent a population at special risk for HCV.[15] Acute HCV infection is typically asymptomatic or characterized by a mild viral syndrome. However, 60% to 70% of infected individuals will go on to develop active liver disease. The use of latex condoms can prevent transmission of HBV and HCV[15] (**Table 8**).

Table 8
Screening, diagnosis, and treatment of hepatitis A, B, and C

			Screening & Diagnosis		
			Screening Frequency		
Virus	Specimen Source	Test	Male	Female	Persons with HIV
HAV	Blood	Hepatitis A IgM	Routine screening not recommended. MSM should be vaccinated if not immune		
HBV	Blood	Hepatitis B surface antigen (HBsAg)	All patients should be screened before initiation of HIV PrEP All adolescents should be vaccinated if not immune		All HIV-infected patients should be tested with HBsAg, hepatitis B core antibody, and hepatitis B surface antibody at entry to care
HCV	Blood	Hepatitis C antibody[a]	Annually if patient has risk factors (MSM or IDU)		Annually or as indicated by risk exposure

	Treatment
Virus	Recommended Regimen
HAV	Supportive care only
HBV	Patients should be referred to a physician with expertise in treatment of hepatitis C
HCV	Patients should be referred to a physician with expertise in treatment of hepatitis C. Consult http://www.hcvguidelines.org for the most up-to-date treatment guidelines

[a] Positive HCV antibody results should be followed with a reflex HCV RNA level.
Data from Workowski KA, Bolan GA, Centers for Disease Control and Prevention. Sexually transmitted diseases treatment guidelines, 2015. MMWR Recomm Rep 2015;64(RR-03):1–137.

Herpes Simplex Viral Infections

Herpes simplex virus (HSV) causes persistent, life-long infection, which most commonly leads to recurrent genital ulcerative disease. Although HSV-1 historically was the cause of oral lesions, and HSV-2 the source of genital lesions, both types are now frequently identified in the oral and genital mucosa. In particular, HSV-1 has been frequently identified in the genital tract of MSM and young women.[15] Adult seroprevalence of HSV-2 is approximately 18% to 22%, with many seroconversions occurring during adolescence.[16,44] Notably, many HSV-seropositive AYA are unaware of their infection.[45] In HSV outbreaks, ulcerative lesions may appear anywhere on the genital, anal, or oral mucosa and are characterized as painful, shallow, and often multiple. They are typically associated with lymphadenopathy that may be bilateral.[46,47] However, many patients may be asymptomatic, even with active lesions, which is the cause of many transmission events. Primary HSV infection may present with a systemic syndrome, including fever, myalgias, headache, and malaise. Recurrent episodes tend to have a milder presentation. Patients should be counseled to avoid sexual contact in the presence of active lesions due to a high degree of viral shedding and because condoms may not cover the entirety of infected mucosa. Although HSV infection is persistent and lifelong, patients may benefit from either episodic treatment at first onset of symptoms, or suppressive therapy with antivirals to reduce symptoms recurrence (**Table 9**).

Table 9
Screening, diagnosis, and treatment of herpes simplex viral infections

Screening & Diagnosis

Specimen Source	Test	Screening Frequency Male	Female	Persons with HIV
Blood	HSV serologies	Asymptomatic screening for HSV with serologies is not recommended due to high population seropositivity		
Lesion	Polymerase chain reaction or cell culture	If lesions present		

Treatment

Site of Infection	Recommended Regimen
First clinical episode of anogenital herpes	• Acyclovir 400 mg po tid × 7–10 d OR • Acyclovir 200 mg po 5 × daily × 7–10 d OR • Valacyclovir 1 g po bid × 7–10 d • Famciclovir 250 mg po tid × 7–10 d
Established infection	Suppressive therapy[a,b,c] • Acyclovir 400 mg po bid[a] OR • Valacyclovir 1 g po daily OR • Valacyclovir 500 mg po daily[b] OR • Famciclovir 250 mg po tid Episodic therapy • Acyclovir 400 mg po tid × 5 d OR • Acyclovir 800 mg po tid × 2 d OR • Valacyclovir 500 mg po bid × 3 d OR • Valacyclovir 1 g po daily × 5 d OR • Famciclovir 1 g po bid × 1 d • Famciclovir 500 mg once followed by 250 mg po bid × 2 d
Patients with HIV	Suppressive therapy • Acyclovir 400–800 mg po bid–tid OR • Valacyclovir 500 mg po bid OR • Famciclovir 500 mg po bid Episodic therapy • Acyclovir 400 mg po tid × 5–10 d OR • Valacyclovir 1 g po daily × 5–10 d OR • Famciclovir 500 mg po bid × 5–10 d
Pregnant women	Suppressive therapy • Acyclovir 400 mg TID

[a] The goal of suppressive therapy is to reduce recurrent symptomatic episodes and/or to reduce sexual transmission. Famciclovir appears somewhat less effective for suppression of viral shedding.
[b] If HSV lesions persist or recur during antiviral treatment, drug resistance should be suspected. Obtaining a viral isolate for sensitivity testing and consulting with an infectious disease expert is recommended.
[c] Valacyclovir 500 mg daily may be less effective than other regimens in patients with very frequent recurrences (≥10/yr).

Data from Workowski KA, Bolan GA, Centers for Disease Control and Prevention. Sexually transmitted diseases treatment guidelines, 2015. MMWR Recomm Rep 2015;64(RR-03):1–137.

Human Papilloma Virus

Human papilloma virus (HPV) causes a wide variety of clinical syndromes in LGBT youth, based on the viral serotype and site of inoculation, including anogenital warts, cervical dysplasia, and anal dysplasia. HPV serotypes 6 and 11 are responsible for an estimated 90% of genital warts or condyloma accuminata.[48] Warts can appear throughout the anogenital region and typically present as skin-colored flat, papillary, or pedunculated lesions with a cauliflower-like appearance. Although these lesions are typically asymptomatic, they may cause itching or burning or may bleed easily when irritated.[49] The oncogenic serotypes 16 to 18 are the chief causes of cervical and anal dysplasia. Risk factors for progression of cervical and anal dysplasia in adolescents include HIV, number of sexual partners, and the presence of external warts.[50] HPV is commonly detected in WSW, and therefore, cervical cancer screening guidelines should follow population guidelines.[7,15,51] Evidence is currently insufficient to recommend routine anal cytology for YMSM to assess for dysplasia.[52,53] For YMSM with HIV, some practices perform yearly cytology with referral to high-resolution anoscopy for any abnormal results (atypical cells of undetermined significance, low-grade squamous intraepithelial lesion, high-grade squamous intraepithelial lesion), but guidelines do not yet recommend routine screening (**Table 10**).[54]

SEXUAL HEALTH COUNSELING AND PREVENTION

Screening for STIs should always be done in concert with preventative counseling. In general, it is best to frame sexual health in a positive preventative health context rather than focusing on fear-based messaging, which may be stigmatizing for youth. AYA should be counseled in how to use latex condoms during sex (oral, anal, and vaginal) to decrease the risk of HIV and STI transmission. In addition to reviewing the mechanics of condom use, discussing sexual health communication and condom negotiation strategies may increase utilization with sex partners.

Human Immunodeficiency Virus Pre-exposure Prophylaxis

HIV prevention has undergone a significant paradigm shift in recent years with the introduction of HIV PrEP. In 2012, the FDA approved the antiretroviral medication tenofovir-emtricitabine (TDF-FTC) as a one-pill-once-daily regimen to be used as part of a comprehensive HIV prevention strategy for adults.[55] In clinical trials of MSM and heterosexual adults, TDF-FTC has been shown to be 44% to 75% effective overall in preventing HIV transmission, and up to 98% effective in those with high levels of medication adherence.[56–58] PrEP is recommended by the CDC, World Health Organization, and US Public Health Service for use as part of a combination HIV prevention strategy in individuals at substantial risk of acquiring HIV.[55,59] Recent data from the IPERGAY trial also suggest that PrEP may be effective when used in an event-driven fashion around sexual activity. The regimen of 2 pills taken 2 to 24 hours before sexual activity and 1 pill at 24 and 48 hours after sexual activity reduced the risk of HIV acquisition by 86%.[24] At this time, however, there are no public health recommendations regarding event driven use.

YMSM and YTW are a key target population for PrEP. However, anyone who is at substantial risk for HIV should be considered candidates for PrEP, including patients with history of STI, multiple sexual partners, HIV serodiscordant partnerships, intravenous (IV) drug use, or transactional sex.[55] Before initiating PrEP, patients must be screened for HIV, because TDF-FTC alone is insufficient for the treatment of HIV and could lead to antiretroviral resistance in patients with undiagnosed infection

Table 10
Screening, diagnosis, and treatment of human papilloma viral infections

Screening & Diagnosis of Cervical and Anal Dysplasia				
Specimen Source	**Test**	**Screening Frequency**		**Persons with HIV**
		Male	**Female**	
Cervix Anus	Cervical cytology via conventional Pap smear or liquid-based cytology (ie, thin prep)[a]	Guidelines not available	Every 3 y for women 21–29	Women should be screened within 1 y of diagnosis and then repeated 6 mo later

Treatment of HPV	
Site of Infection	**Recommended Regimen**

External anogenital wart	Patient-applied
	• Imiquimod 5% cream[b,c]
	   OR
	• Podofilox 0.5% solution or gel[b]
	   OR
	• Sinecatechins 15% ointment[b]
	Provider-administered
	• Cryotherapy with liquid nitrogen or cryoprobe[d]
	   OR
	• Trichloroacetic acid (TCA) 80%–90%
	   OR
	• Bichloroacetic acid (BCA) 80%–90%
	   OR
	• Surgical removal (scissor excision, tangential shave excision, curettage, laser or electrosurgery)

Mucosal genital warts[e]	• Cryotherapy
	   OR
	• TCA or BCA 80%–90%
	   OR
	• Surgical removal

[a] HPV co-testing not recommended in women <30 years of age.
[b] Safety in pregnancy has not been established; pregnancy category C.
[c] May weaken latex condoms and diaphragms.
[d] Do not use cryoprobe in vagina because or risk of perforation or fistula.
[e] Cervical and intra-anal warts should be managed in consultation with specialist.
   Data from Workowski KA, Bolan GA, Centers for Disease Control and Prevention. Sexually transmitted diseases treatment guidelines, 2015. MMWR Recomm Rep 2015;64(RR-03):1–137.

(**Table 11**). Finally, PrEP is meant to be used as part of a combination prevention strategy along with condom promotion, partner communication, and regular HIV and STI testing. It is important for patients to understand that it takes an estimated 7 days for PrEP to reach peak efficacy in the rectal mucosa and closer to 3 weeks in the vaginal mucosa, and protective levels wane quickly during adherence lapses. If patients have a positive HIV test while taking PrEP, TDF-FTC should be immediately discontinued and confirmatory HIV testing should be sent. Additional guidance on PrEP provision is available from the US Public Health Service at http://www.cdc.gov/hiv/pdf/prepguidelines2014.pdf.[55]

Table 11
Human immunodeficiency virus pre-exposure prophylaxis laboratory tests and visit schedule

	Baseline Visit	Every 3 mo (Minimum)	Every 6 mo (Minimum)
HIV testing[a]	X	X	–
Assess for symptoms of AHI[b]	X	X	–
Hepatitis B surface antigen,[c] hepatitis C serology	X	–	–
Hepatitis B immunization if nonimmune	X	–	–
Serum creatinine[d]	X	–	X
STI testing	X	–	X (at minimum)
Pregnancy testing	X	X	–
Assess for side effects[e]	–	X	–
Adherence counseling	X	X	–
Prevention counseling	X	X	–

[a] Rapid or fourth-generation assay, send HIV RNA qualitative or quantitative if concern for high-risk recent exposure with last month, or if symptoms of AHI.
[b] Typically fever, rash, pharyngitis, lymphadenopathy. If present within preceding month, send HIV RNA qualitative or quantitative assay to rule out HIV infection.
[c] Patients with positive HBSAg should be evaluated by a clinician experienced in treatment of HBV before initiating PrEP. TDF-FTC is also used to treat hepatitis B, and abrupt discontinuation in patients with HBV can cause fulminant liver failure.
[d] TDF-FTC is contraindicated if creatinine clearance less than 60 mL/min because it has known nephrotoxic potential.
[e] Most commonly nausea, GI upset, and headache.
   Data from US Public Health Service. Preexposure prophylaxis for the prevention of HIV infection in the United States–2014 clinical practice guideline. Centers for Disease Control and Prevention, Department of Health and Human Services. Atlanta (GA): US Public Health Service; 2014. p. 1–67.

Human Immunodeficiency Virus Postexposure Prophylaxis

Although PrEP is a highly effective and long-term means of preventing HIV before exposure occurs, HIV postexposure prophylaxis (PEP) can prevent transmission in the setting of an acute exposure. Data on the efficacy of nonoccupational PEP are limited and are drawn largely from observational cohort studies of patients after sexual assault and on data from the use of occupational PEP to prevent transmission.[60] However, the routine use of occupational PEP to prevent health care workplace exposures has resulted in a dramatic decrease of reported occupational transmissions, with only one reported transmission since 1999.[61] Nonoccupational PEP, as recommended by the CDC, consists of 3 antiretroviral medications of at least 2 classes given for a fixed time interval of 28 days. Timing is an essential aspect of PEP provision and should be initiated as close as possible to the time of HIV exposure, and not after 72 hours. In general, PEP should be recommended in cases of unprotected receptive or insertive vaginal or anal intercourse, needle sharing, or blood or potentially infected fluid exposure where the source is HIV infected or of unknown HIV status (**Fig. 2**).[60,62,63] PEP should be considered on a case-by-case basis for lower-risk exposures, including oral-vaginal, oral-penile, or oral-anal contact. Factors to consider in these cases, which could increase the risk of HIV transmission, include untreated HIV and high viral load in the source patient, the presence of nonintact mucosa or genital trauma in both partners, and the presence of concurrent STI in both partners.[63] In cases where expert consultation is needed to determine the need for PEP, clinicians can consult the 24-hour National Clinicians' Consultation Center PEPline at 1-888-448-4911.

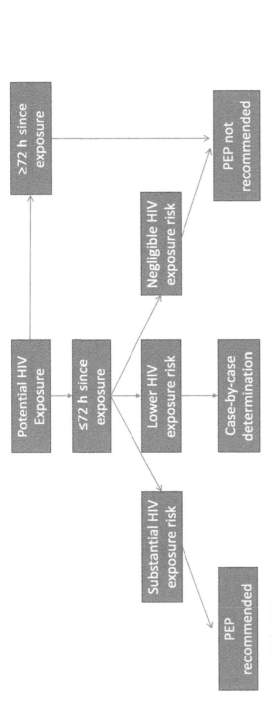

Substantial Risk for HIV Exposure:

Receptive and insertive vaginal or anal intercourse

Needle sharing

Blood or bloody-fluid exposure to mucous membrane

OR

Lower-risk exposure in setting of HIV-infected source with high viral load, nonintact mucosa, or genital ulcer disease or STI

When:

The source is known to be HIV-infected or HIV status unknown

Lower Risk for HIV Exposure:

Receptive or insertive oral-vaginal, oral-anal, or oral-penile contact

When:

The source is known to be HIV-infected or HIV status unknown

Negligible Risk for HIV Exposure

Oral-oral contact without mucosal damage

Human bites not involving blood

Mutual masturbation without skin breakdown

Regardless:

Of the known or suspected HIV status of the source

Fig. 2. Algorithm for evaluation for HIV PEP. (*Adapted from* Kuhar, DT, Henderson DK, Struble KA, et al. Updated US Public Health Service guidelines for the management of occupational exposures to human immunodeficiency virus and recommendations for postexposure prophylaxis. Infect Control Hosp Epidemiol 2013;34(9):875–92; and New York State Department of Public Health. HIV prophylaxis after non-occupational exposure. 2013. Available at: http://hivguidelines.org/clinical-guidelines/post-exposure-prophylaxis/hiv-prophylaxis-following-non-occupational-exposure/. Accessed August 12, 2016.)

Before initiating PEP, the exposed patient needs HIV testing to rule out undiagnosed HIV infection at baseline as well as testing for pregnancy, renal and hepatic function, and hepatitis status. However, the initiation of PEP should not be delayed while waiting for results, because efficacy decreases with time from exposure. The current recommended PEP regimen is once-daily TDF-FTC and twice-daily raltegravir given together for 28 days. TDF-FTC should not be used in the setting of renal impairment, for patients less than 13 years of age, or those with a Tanner stage less than 3. Alternate regimens are available, and for additional guidance on PEP provision, physicians can contact the National Clinicians' Consultation Center PEPline.[60,62,63] Exposed patients should be followed frequently while on PEP, and follow-up HIV testing should be performed at 4 to 6 weeks and 12 weeks after the initial exposure with a fourth-generation antigen/antibody assay (**Table 12**). Patients with a history of repeated PEP use should receive counseling on starting PrEP.[61,64]

Immunizations

In addition to condoms and HIV chemoprophylaxis, routine vaccination is a highly effective preventative health measure against HAV, HBV, and HPV. The quadrivalent HPV vaccine is recommended for all women ages 11 to 26 and men ages 11 to 21 to prevent high-risk HPV vaccination with HPV types 6, 11, 16, and 18. As MSM are at high risk of HPV-associated anal lesions and progression to anal dysplasia, HPV vaccination is routinely recommended through age 26 for MSM and men living with HIV.[15] The Advisory Committee on Immunization Practices now recommends the recently licensed 9-valent HPV vaccine, which includes 5 additional cancer-associated types (31, 33, 45, 52, and 58).[65] Routine HPV vaccination has resulted in population level decreases in both oncogenic and nononcogenic strain HPV prevalence, and reduced rates of anal dysplasia in MSM.[66,67] For minor youth, when parents

Table 12
Human immunodeficiency virus postexposure prophylaxis visit and laboratory testing schedule

	Baseline	Week 1	Week 2	Week 3	Week 4	Week 12
Clinic visit	X	X w/in 72 h[f]	X	X Or phone	X	X
HIV testing of exposed patient[a]	X	–	–	–	X	X
Pregnancy testing[b]	X	–	X	–	–	–
Renal and hepatic function testing[c]	X	–	X	–	X	–
STI testing[d]	X	–	X	–	–	–
Hepatitis B Surface Antigen[e]	X	–	–	–	–	X
Hepatitis C Antibody	X	–	–	–	–	X

[a] Preferably with fourth-generation assay. If symptoms of AHI or high-risk encounter in proceeding 6 weeks, test with qualitative or quantitative HIV RNA. Every attempt should be made to test the source patient as well and PEP can be discontinued if the source has a negative fourth-generation test with no symptoms of acute HIV or high-risk exposures in preceding 6 wk.
[b] Consider emergency contraception if unprotected intercourse in previous 96 h.
[c] TDF-FTC is contraindicated in patients with renal impairment.
[d] Gonorrhea, chlamydia, and syphilis. In cases of sexual assault or if concern for STI coinfection, treat empirically with ceftriaxone, azithromycin, and metronidazole.
[e] Immunize against hepatitis B if not previously immunized.
[f] To assess side effects (typically nausea, vomiting, headache) and adherence.
Data from Refs.[60,62,63]

or guardians are present at clinic visits, targeting vaccine messaging around preventative health benefits may increase uptake.[68] Finally, for all AYA, and MSM in particular, hepatitis vaccination can reduce potential morbidity associated with HAV and HBV, and patients should be caught up if not fully immunized.

FAMILY PLANNING

Another important aspect of providing sexual health care for LGBT youth involves discussing current and future family planning intentions. Providers should not make assumptions about pregnancy or fertility intensions or prevention among LGBT youth. Although some WSW may have never had male sexual contact, the majority (53%–97%) have previously had male partners, with 5% to 28% reporting male partners in the past year.[15,69] In addition, LGBT youth are no less likely to plan for parenthood, and inquiring about family planning intentions allows providers another opportunity to better understand how patients visualize their futures and sense of family. For youth living with HIV, family planning conversations may be an opportunity to introduce discussion of PrEP for serodiscordant partners.

Providing safe and effective contraception is an essential preventative health task for youth at risk of pregnancy. When discussing methods, providers should start discussion with the long-acting reversible contraceptive methods, because they are the most efficacious.[51] With contraceptive efficacy of greater than 99% with both perfect and typical use, the intrauterine devices (IUDs) and contraceptive implant (Nexplanon) are top-tier choices for AYA.[51] Utilization of IUDs has historically been low in adolescents, due both to access issues and to provider concerns regarding perceived associated risk of PID. In fact, the rate of PID in IUD users is low, and this risk can be essentially eliminated by screening for gonorrhea and chlamydia at the time of insertion. In addition, the contraceptive implant is a slow-release progestin–based device that is inserted into the upper arm and can provide 3 years of highly effective contraception.[51,70–72]

Injectable medroxyprogesterone acetate (Depo Provera), combined hormonal oral contraceptives, contraceptive patch, and contraceptive ring, although less efficacious (typical use efficacy 91%–94%), may be more attractive to youth who do not want to commit to long-term method use. For transgender men, Depo Provera, continuously cycled combined hormonal contraceptives, and progestin-based IUDs (Mirena, Skyla) are all effective options for menstrual suppression as well. It is also important to note that for transmen-identified youth who are on GnRH agonists or masculinizing hormone therapy (testosterone), these medications may not completely suppress ovulation and may be teratogenic, and therefore, additional contraceptive options may be required. Before prescribing contraception, patient and family past medical histories should be reviewed for any comorbidities that may affect method selection (ie, personal or family history of coagulopathy for estrogen-based methods). In addition, medications should be reviewed for interactions that may decrease contraceptive efficacy, such as ART.[72]

Counseling for all methods should emphasize the importance of ongoing condom use to prevent HIV and STIs. In addition, discussion and provision of emergency contraception in the form of levonorgestrol (Plan B) or ulipristal acetate (Ella) can reduce the risk of unintended pregnancy after unprotected sex. When taken within 96 hours, these methods can significantly reduce unintended pregnancy, with failure rates of 0.9% to 2.1% for ulipristal and 0.6% to 3.1% for levonorgestrol, respectively. Advance provision of emergency contraception increases the likelihood of use in the event of unprotected intercourse, without increasing sexual risk behavior.[73–75]

Additional guidance on contraceptive method selection and usage can be found through the US Medical Eligibility Criteria for Contraceptive Use http://www.cdc.gov/reproductivehealth/unintendedpregnancy/usmec.htm, as well as the US Selected Practice Recommendations (US SPR) for Contraceptive Use http://www.cdc.gov/reproductivehealth/unintendedpregnancy/usspr.htm.

For LGBT youth who have only same sex partners or who may have impaired fertility due to gender-affirming treatments, providers should not make assumptions about desires for childbearing, because LGBT youth may have needs for family planning similar to their cisgender and heterosexual counterparts. Childbearing options include assisted reproductive technologies, surrogacy, and adoption, and referrals to appropriate subspecialists may be made.[76–78] Specifically, for transgender youth considering gender-affirming hormone therapy, understanding family planning intentions is essential before proceeding with hormones because both feminizing and masculinizing therapies may irreversibly impair fertility. Fertility-preserving options, including oocyte cryopreservation and sperm banking, may be available, but must be undertaken after puberty and before starting cross-gender hormones (for further discussion, see Annelou L.C. de Vries and colleagues' article, "What the Primary Care Pediatrician Needs to Know about Gender Incongruence and Gender Dysphoria in Children and Adolescents," in this issue).[79] Also, although some assume that taking testosterone will prevent pregnancy, there are reports of cases of pregnancy among people either on or who have recently stopped testosterone.

SUMMARY

Health care providers can make a critical impact on the lives of LGBT patients by providing supportive, comprehensive sexual and reproductive health care. Counseling youth on sexual development, screening for and treating STIs, diagnosing HIV and linking youth to care, providing sexual health preventative care such as vaccines and PrEP, and delivering reproductive health care including contraception are all ways providers can improve individual patient outcomes, while also creating substantial public health benefit. By offering youth-centered, gender- and sexuality-affirming sexual health services, providers can begin to mitigate many of the health care inequities faced by LGBT youth.

REFERENCES

1. Mustanski B, Van Wagenen A, Birkett M, et al. Identifying sexual orientation health disparities in adolescents: analysis of pooled data from the Youth Risk Behavior Survey, 2005 and 2007. Am J Public Health 2014;104(2):211–7.
2. Link B, Phelan JC, Hatzenbuehler ML. The role of stigma in the production and maintenance of inequality. In: McLeod J, Lawler E, Schwalbe M, editors. Handbook of the social psychology of inequality. New York: Springer; 2014. p. 49–64.
3. Conron KJ, Mimiaga MJ, Landers SJ. A population-based study of sexual orientation identity and gender differences in adult health. Am J Public Health 2010; 100(10):1953–60.
4. Kann L, Olsen EO, McManus T, et al. Sexual identity, sex of sexual contacts, and health-risk behaviors among students in grades 9-12–youth risk behavior surveillance, selected sites, United States, 2001-2009. MMWR Surveill Summ 2011; 60(7):1–133.
5. Benson PA, Hergenroeder AC. Bacterial sexually transmitted infections in gay, lesbian, and bisexual adolescents: medical and public health perspectives. Semin Pediatr Infect Dis 2005;16(3):181–91.

6. Purcell DW, Johnson CH, Lansky A, et al. Estimating the population size of men who have sex with men in the United States to obtain HIV and syphilis rates. Open AIDS J 2012;6:98–107.

7. Agwu AL, Neptune A, Voss C, et al. CD4 counts of nonperinatally HIV-infected youth and young adults presenting for HIV care between 2002 and 2010. JAMA Pediatr 2014;168(4):381–3.

8. CDC. HIV Among Transgender People in the United States. 2013.

9. Millett GA, Peterson JL, Flores SA, et al. Comparisons of disparities and risks of HIV infection in black and other men who have sex with men in Canada, UK, and USA: a meta-analysis. Lancet 2012;380(9839):341–8.

10. Lindley LL, Walsemann KM. Sexual orientation and risk of pregnancy among New York City high-school students. Am J Public Health 2015;105(7):1379–86.

11. Guttmacher Institute. State Policies in Brief: Minors' Access to STI Services 2015.

12. Ginsburg K, Kinsman S. Reaching teens: strength based communication strategies to build resilience and support healthy adolescent development. Elk Grove Village (IL): American Academy of Pediatrics; 2014.

13. Kaiser Permanente National Diversity council. A provider's handbook on culturally competent care. 2nd edition. Oakland (CA): Kaiser Foundation Health Plan Inc; 2004.

14. Chandra A, Mosher WD, Copen C, et al. Sexual behavior, sexual attraction, and sexual identity in the United States: data from the 2006-2008 National Survey of Family Growth. Natl Health Stat Report 2011;(36):1–36.

15. Workowski KA, Bolan GA, Centers for Disease Control and Prevention. Sexually transmitted diseases treatment guidelines, 2015. MMWR Recomm Rep 2015; 64(RR-03):1–137.

16. Centers for Disease Control and Prevention. Sexually Transmitted Disease Surveillance, 2013. Atlanta (GA); 2014.

17. Paz-Bailey G, Sternberg M, Puren AJ, et al. Determinants of HIV type 1 shedding from genital ulcers among men in South Africa. Clin Infect Dis 2010;50(7):1060–7.

18. Centers for Disease C. HIV among youth. 2010.

19. Zanoni BC, Mayer KH. The adolescent and young adult HIV cascade of care in the United States: exaggerated health disparities. AIDS Patient Care STDS 2014;28(3):128–35.

20. Kahn JO, Walker BD. Acute human immunodeficiency virus type 1 infection. N Engl J Med 1998;339(1):33–9.

21. McKellar MS, Cope AB, Gay CL, et al. Acute HIV-1 infection in the Southeastern United States: a cohort study. AIDS Res Hum Retroviruses 2013;29(1):121–8.

22. Committee on Pediatric AIDS, Emmanuel PJ, Martinez J, et al. Adolescents and HIV infection: the pediatrician's role in promoting routine testing. Pediatrics 2011; 128(5):1023–9.

23. Centers for Disease Control and Prevention (CDC). National HIV Testing Day and new testing recommendations. MMWR Morb Mortal Wkly Rep 2014;63(25):537.

24. Molina JM, Capitant C, Spire B, et al. On-demand preexposure prophylaxis in men at high risk for HIV-1 infection. N Engl J Med 2015;373(23):2237–46.

25. Cheret A, Bacchus-Souffan C, Avettand-Fenoel V, et al. Combined ART started during acute HIV infection protects central memory CD4+ T cells and can induce remission. J Antimicrob Chemother 2015;70(7):2108–20.

26. Pinsky L, Chiarilli DB, Klausner JD, et al. Rates of asymptomatic nonurethral gonorrhea and chlamydia in a population of university men who have sex with men. J Am Coll Health 2012;60(6):481–4.

27. Park J, Marcus JL, Pandori M, et al. Sentinel surveillance for pharyngeal chlamydia and gonorrhea among men who have sex with men–San Francisco, 2010. Sex Transm Dis 2012;39(6):482–4.

28. Singh D, Fine DN, Marrazzo JM. Chlamydia trachomatis infection among women reporting sexual activity with women screened in Family Planning Clinics in the Pacific Northwest, 1997 to 2005. Am J Public Health 2011;101(7):1284–90.

29. Scholes D, Stergachis A, Heidrich FE, et al. Prevention of pelvic inflammatory disease by screening for cervical chlamydial infection. N Engl J Med 1996;334(21): 1362–6.

30. Craib KJ, Meddings DR, Strathdee SA, et al. Rectal gonorrhoea as an independent risk factor for HIV infection in a cohort of homosexual men. Genitourin Med 1995;71(3):150–4.

31. Centers for Disease Control and Prevention. Sexually Transmitted Disease Surveillance U.S. Department of Health and Human Services, 2004. 2003.

32. Kellock D, O'Mahony CP. Sexually acquired metronidazole-resistant trichomoniasis in a lesbian couple. Genitourin Med 1996;72(1):60–1.

33. Deguchi T, Yasuda M, Ito S. Management of pharyngeal gonorrhea is crucial to prevent the emergence and spread of antibiotic-resistant Neisseria gonorrhoeae. Antimicrob Agents Chemother 2012;56(7):4039–40 [author reply: 4041–2].

34. Morris M, Nicoll A, Simms I, et al. Bacterial vaginosis: a public health review. BJOG 2001;108(5):439–50.

35. Fethers KA, Fairley CK, Hocking JS, et al. Sexual risk factors and bacterial vaginosis: a systematic review and meta-analysis. Clin Infect Dis 2008;47(11): 1426–35.

36. Evans AL, Scally AJ, Wellard SJ, et al. Prevalence of bacterial vaginosis in lesbians and heterosexual women in a community setting. Sex Transm Infect 2007;83(6):470–5.

37. Berger BJ, Kolton S, Zenilman JM, et al. Bacterial vaginosis in lesbians: a sexually transmitted disease. Clin Infect Dis 1995;21(6):1402–5.

38. Marrazzo JM, Koutsky LA, Eschenbach DA, et al. Characterization of vaginal flora and bacterial vaginosis in women who have sex with women. J Infect Dis 2002; 185(9):1307–13.

39. Marrazzo JM, Thomas KK, Fiedler TL, et al. Risks for acquisition of bacterial vaginosis among women who report sex with women: a cohort study. PLoS One 2010;5(6):e11139.

40. Marrazzo JM, Thomas KK, Ringwood K. A behavioural intervention to reduce persistence of bacterial vaginosis among women who report sex with women: results of a randomised trial. Sex Transm Infect 2011;87(5):399–405.

41. Kelley CF, Rosenberg ES, O'Hara BM, et al. Prevalence of urethral Trichomonas vaginalis in black and white men who have sex with men. Sex Transm Dis 2012; 39(9):739.

42. McClelland RS, Sangare L, Hassan WM, et al. Infection with Trichomonas vaginalis increases the risk of HIV-1 acquisition. J Infect Dis 2007;195(5):698–702.

43. Moodley P, Wilkinson D, Connolly C, et al. Trichomonas vaginalis is associated with pelvic inflammatory disease in women infected with human immunodeficiency virus. Clin Infect Dis 2002;34(4):519–22.

44. Oster AM, Sternberg M, Nebenzahl S, et al. Prevalence of HIV, sexually transmitted infections, and viral hepatitis by Urbanicity, among men who have sex with men, injection drug users, and heterosexuals in the United States. Sex Transm Dis 2014;41(4):272–9.

45. Schulte JM, Bellamy AR, Hook EW 3rd, et al. HSV-1 and HSV-2 seroprevalence in the United States among asymptomatic women unaware of any herpes simplex virus infection (Herpevac Trial for Women). South Med J 2014;107(2):79–84.

46. Workowski KA. Skin and mucous membrane infections and inguinal lymphadenopathy. In: Long SS, editor. Principles and practice of pediatric infectious diseases. 4th edition. Philadelphia: Elsevier; 2012. p. 349–52.

47. Chayavichitsilp P, Buckwalter JV, Krakowski AC, et al. Herpes simplex. Pediatr Rev 2009;30(4):119–29 [quiz: 130].

48. Garland SM, Steben M, Sings HL, et al. Natural history of genital warts: analysis of the placebo arm of 2 randomized phase III trials of a quadrivalent human papillomavirus (types 6, 11, 16, and 18) vaccine. J Infect Dis 2009;199(6):805–14.

49. Sinclair KA, Woods CR, Sinal SH. Venereal warts in children. Pediatr Rev 2011; 32(3):115–21 [quiz: 121].

50. Moscicki AB, Durako SJ, Houser J, et al. Human papillomavirus infection and abnormal cytology of the anus in HIV-infected and uninfected adolescents. AIDS 2003;17(3):311–20.

51. Committee on Adolescent Health Care Long-Acting Reversible Contraception Working Group, The American College of Obstetricians and Gynecologists. Committee opinion no. 539: adolescents and long-acting reversible contraception: implants and intrauterine devices. Obstet Gynecol 2012;120(4):983–8.

52. Machalek DA, Poynten M, Jin F, et al. Anal human papillomavirus infection and associated neoplastic lesions in men who have sex with men: a systematic review and meta-analysis. Lancet Oncol 2012;13(5):487–500.

53. Salit IE, Lytwyn A, Raboud J, et al. The role of cytology (Pap tests) and human papillomavirus testing in anal cancer screening. AIDS 2010;24(9):1307–13.

54. Panel on Opportunistic Infections in HIV-Infected Adults and Adolescents. Guidelines for the prevention and treatment of opportunistic infections in HIV-infected adults and adolescents: recommendations from the Centers for Disease Control and Prevention, the National Institutes of Health, and the HIV Medicine Association of the Infectious Diseases Society of America. 2015.

55. US Public Health Service. Preexposure prophylaxis for the prevention of HIV infection in the United States–2014 clinical practice guideline. Centers for Disease Control and Prevention, Department of Health and Human Services. Atlanta (GA): US Public Health Service; 2014. p. 1–67.

56. Baeten JM, Donnell D, Ndase P, et al. Antiretroviral prophylaxis for HIV prevention in heterosexual men and women. N Engl J Med 2012;367(5):399–410.

57. Grant RM, Lama JR, Anderson PL, et al. Preexposure chemoprophylaxis for HIV prevention in men who have sex with men. N Engl J Med 2010;363(27):2587–99.

58. Grant RM, Anderson PL, McMahan V, et al. Uptake of pre-exposure prophylaxis, sexual practices, and HIV incidence in men and transgender women who have sex with men: a cohort study. Lancet Infect Dis 2014;14(9):820–9.

59. World Health Organization. Guideline on when to start antiretroviral therapy and on preexposure prophylaxis for HIV. 2015:1–78.

60. Smith DK, Grohskopf LA, Black RJ, et al. Antiretroviral postexposure prophylaxis after sexual, injection-drug use, or other nonoccupational exposure to HIV in the United States: recommendations from the U.S. Department of Health and Human Services. MMWR Recomm Rep 2005;54(RR-2):1–20.

61. United States Public Health Service. Pre-exposure prophylaxis for the prevention of HIV infection—2014: a clinical practice guideline 2014.

62. Kuhar DT, Henderson DK, Struble KA, et al. Updated US Public Health Service guidelines for the management of occupational exposures to human

immunodeficiency virus and recommendations for postexposure prophylaxis. Infect Control Hosp Epidemiol 2013;34(9):875–92.

63. New York State Department of Public Health. HIV prophylaxis after non-occupational exposure 2013. Available at: http://www.hivguidelines.org/clinical-guidelines/post-exposure-prophylaxis/hiv-prophylaxis-following-non-occupational-exposure/. Accessed August 12, 2016.

64. Marrazzo JM, del Rio C, Holtgrave DR, et al. HIV prevention in clinical care settings: 2014 recommendations of the International Antiviral Society-USA Panel. JAMA 2014;312(4):390–409.

65. Petrosky E, Bocchini JA Jr, Hariri S, et al. Use of 9-valent human papillomavirus (HPV) vaccine: updated HPV vaccination recommendations of the advisory committee on immunization practices. MMWR Morb Mortal Wkly Rep 2015;64(11): 300–4.

66. Drolet M, Benard E, Boily MC, et al. Population-level impact and herd effects following human papillomavirus vaccination programmes: a systematic review and meta-analysis. Lancet Infect Dis 2015;15(5):565–80.

67. Centers for Disease Control and Prevention. Vital signs: HIV infection, testing, and risk behaviors among youths—United States. MMWR Morb Mortal Wkly Rep 2012;61(47):971–6.

68. Gainforth HL, Cao W, Latimer-Cheung AE. Message framing and parents' intentions to have their children vaccinated against HPV. Public Health Nurs 2012; 29(6):542–52.

69. Marrazzo JM, Stine K. Reproductive health history of lesbians: implications for care. Am J Obstet Gynecol 2004;190(5):1298–304.

70. Division of Reproductive Health, National Center for Chronic Disease Prevention and Health Promotion, Centers for Disease Control and Prevention (CDC). U.S. selected practice recommendations for contraceptive use, 2013: adapted from the World Health Organization selected practice recommendations for contraceptive use, 2nd edition. MMWR Morb Mortal Wkly Rep 2013;62(RR–05):1–61.

71. Russo JA, Miller E, Gold MA. Myths and misconceptions about long-acting reversible contraception (LARC). J Adolesc Health 2013;52(4 Suppl):S14–21.

72. Centers for Disease Control and Prevention (CDC). US. medical eligibility criteria for contraceptive use, 2010. MMWR Recomm Rep 2010;59(RR-4):1–86.

73. Gold MA. In support of emergency contraception. J Pediatr Adolesc Gynecol 1999;12(4):229–30.

74. Raine TR, Harper CC, Rocca CH, et al. Direct access to emergency contraception through pharmacies and effect on unintended pregnancy and STIs: a randomized controlled trial. JAMA 2005;293(1):54–62.

75. Stewart HE, Gold MA, Parker AM. The impact of using emergency contraception on reproductive health outcomes: a retrospective review in an urban adolescent clinic. J Pediatr Adolesc Gynecol 2003;16(5):313–8.

76. Greenfeld DA, Seli E. Gay men choosing parenthood through assisted reproduction: medical and psychosocial considerations. Fertil Steril 2011;95(1):225–9.

77. Norton W, Hudson N, Culley L. Gay men seeking surrogacy to achieve parenthood. Reprod Biomed Online 2013;27(3):271–9.

78. von Doussa H, Power J, Riggs D. Imagining parenthood: the possibilities and experiences of parenthood among transgender people. Cult Health Sex 2015;17(9): 1119–31.

79. World Professional Association for Transgender Health. Standards of care for the health of transsexual, transgender, and gender-nonconforming people, Seventh Edition. Int J Transgend 2012;13(4):165–232.

Substance Abuse Prevention, Assessment, and Treatment for Lesbian, Gay, Bisexual, and Transgender Youth

Romulo Alcalde Aromin Jr, MD

KEYWORDS

• LGBT • Substance abuse • Assessment • Youth • Prevention programs

KEY POINTS

- There are limited data on the epidemiology of drug use among gay, lesbian, bisexual, and transgender youth; its prevalence is inferred from field studies.
- Preventive programs foster skill building, general wellness, and specific refusal skills; The success of preventive programs hinges on community "buyin."
- The Screening, Brief Intervention, Referral and Treatment should be part of routine examination to identify those at more serious risks requiring a more targeted assessment and treatment.
- Incorporating gender and sexual orientation issues into treatment that works enhances engagement and retention. When indicated, medications should be considered and supported.

INTRODUCTION

Knowing how to manage substance abuse in all youth is an important aspect of pediatric care, including providing clinically appropriate anticipatory guidance, monitoring, assessment, and treatment. Although most lesbian, gay, bisexual, and transgender (LGBT) youth do not abuse substances, as a group they experience unique challenges in self-identity development[1] that put them at somewhat of an increased risk for substance abuse. This article addresses the prevention and management of substance use in LGBT youth relevant to clinical practice in pediatrics and allied professions as an aspect of their overall health care. It reviews basic information about substance abuse in youth and discusses special considerations relevant to LGBT youth.

The author has nothing to disclose.
Psychiatry, Psychosocial Services, Institute for Family Health, 16E 16th St, New York, NY 10003, USA
E-mail address: raarominjr@yahoo.com

Pediatr Clin N Am 63 (2016) 1057–1077
http://dx.doi.org/10.1016/j.pcl.2016.07.007
0031-3955/16/© 2016 Elsevier Inc. All rights reserved.

EPIDEMIOLOGY

A number of national epidemiologic surveys monitor substance use among youth in the United States (available: www.monitoringthefuture.org[2]); the National Survey on Drug Use and Health (available: https://nsduhweb.rti.org/[3]); the Youth Risk Behavior Surveillance System: biennial Centers for Disease Control Survey (available: www.cdc.gov/healthyyouth/yrbs/index.htm[4]), although these have not monitored routinely in LGBT youth specifically. The epidemiology of drug use among LGBT youth needs to be studied further. Dimensions on sexual orientation (sexual identity, sexual attraction, and sexual behavior) should be incorporated as each confers differential drug use profile.[5] Subsequent trends can then be followed meaningfully and contrasted with heterosexual youth.

However, some data do exist on the epidemiology of substance use among this group. A community-based cohort of US adolescents were surveyed from 1999 to 2005 looking at whether minority sexual orientation is a risk for drug use.[6] Respondents whose sexual orientation was mostly heterosexual, bisexual, or lesbian/gay were more likely than completely heterosexual youth to report past-year illicit drug use and misuse of prescription drugs. Further, bisexual females were most likely to report use. Age was also considered significant with larger use during adolescence compared with early adulthood. In this study, the prevalence of drug use was much higher when compared with respondents in the 2002 National Survey of Drug Use and Health. Marijuana is the most prevalent drug of abuse. Other studies replicated these results.[7] Drug use has been found to accelerate more quickly over time among LGBT youth compared with heterosexual youth.[8] There is also increased prevalence of methamphetamine[9] and alcohol use and binge drinking among young men who have sex with men.[10]

Risk Factors for Substance Abuse

Research has demonstrated a number of risk and protective factors in youth for developing substance abuse. These allow clinicians to identify risks for drug use early on, and to monitor those youth at risk appropriately. They include:

1. Difficult temperament,
2. Reduced attention span,
3. Irritability,
4. Externalizing behavior (acting out of anger), and
5. Genetic factors (twin studies indicate 40%–60% heritability of risk).

Alcoholism onset before age 25 is more likely in those who are male and aggressive (with or without alcohol use), display high novelty seeking, low harm avoidance, and are not motivated by rewards.

In addition to the general risk factors for substance use in youth described, additional risk factors include feelings of being "different" and alienated for the LGBT youth. Bias-motivated bullying victimization, which is highly prevalent among LGBT youth (see Valerie A. Earnshaw and colleagues' article, "LGBT Youth and Bullying," in this issue), is associated with high-risk sexual behaviors (unprotected anal sexual intercourse, sometimes with concomitant drug use), and increases the risk of infection with the human immunodeficiency virus (HIV) among sexual minority youth. Young racial minority men who have sex with men are at especially increased risk of HIV infection. Internalized homonegativity is also found to be associated with drug use.[11–15] Fortunately, there is evidence that, as sexual minority youth transition to early adulthood, victimization can decrease (It Gets Better Project).[16] This underscores the importance of protecting LGBT youth affected by a nexus of adverse sociocultural factors like interpersonal and self-stigma, epidemic problems like HIV, and mental health needs that may include substance abuse during a developmental period when they may be at heightened risk.

Social media is an important aspect of peer relationships for contemporary youth, with experiences that may both heighten and mitigate risk. Although social media can lead to the advent of phenomena such as cyberbullying, online friends can be important novel sources of social support, particularly for LGBT youth.[17] Having a drug-using friend is a significant factor contributing to initiating and continuing substance use.

Protective Factors for Substance Abuse

Protective factors modify the effect of exposure to stressful life events to decrease the likelihood of developing substance abuse.[18] These include:

1. Parent engagement with youth, such as spending time with them, ensuring reliable "family time" on weekends, and being emotionally available.
2. Positive parenting practices such as appropriate (neither lax nor overly harsh and arbitrary) discipline, fostering positive behaviors, having positive attitudes toward an LBGT child, and having appropriate discussions with teens about sex, intimacy, relationships, and the prevention of HIV, STDs, and pregnancy.
3. "School connectedness" – that is, a positive feeling toward school, being less likely to engage in risk behaviors, and having better academic functioning.

NEUROBIOLOGY OF DRUG ABUSE

Substance abuse is related to activity in specific brain regions. This includes a "reward circuit" of dopaminergic neurons in the ventral tegmental area that communicate to the nucleus accumbens, which then communicates to the cortex.[19] Drugs of abuse are active in these brain regions, either mimicking the effects neurotransmitters (eg, heroin and lysergic acid diethylamide), blocking transmission (eg, phencyclidine), blocking synaptic reuptake (eg, cocaine) with net increase in presynaptic cells, or increasing release of neurotransmitters (methamphetamine).

Although biologically mediated, drug-seeking behavior is best understood in the context of its environment. Understanding that drug use or relapse can be triggered by environmental cues that precede use is key in identifying high-risk situations and learning new coping skills through alternative, non–drug-seeking behaviors.

GATEWAY DRUGS

The gateway hypothesis posits that tobacco or alcohol use sets the stage for subsequent marijuana and other illicit drug use. Consistent with this hypothesis, younger onset and increased frequency of use predict progression.[20] In an animal model, nicotine potentiates subsequent cocaine exposure involving the amygdala, one of the structures implicated in drug use.[21] Below is information on substances that are more likely to be used by LGBT youth and hypothesized to act as gateway drugs.

Nicotine

White LGBT individuals are more likely than the general population to use tobacco products, including smoked tobacco and electronic cigarettes. There is also an increased likelihood of nicotine use in sexual minority youth,[22] especially bisexual girls,[23] compared with heterosexuals. Unique factors associated with tobacco use in LGBT youth include limited socialization, stress, and a desire to project masculinity in males, and may suggest specific approaches to smoking prevention and cessation relevant to LGBT youth.[24–26]

Alcohol

Between 2001 and 2005, 4700 youth younger than 21 years of age died as a result of alcohol. Alcohol binges, defined as more than 5 drinks in males and more than 4 in females, within 2 hours, bringing the blood alcohol level to 0.08 g % or higher, is a typical pattern of abuse in adolescents. This can result in blackouts and alcohol poisoning. Most teens have their first drink in June or July. Teen drivers are at 3-fold risk greater of being in a fatal vehicular accident. To appreciate equivalents of alcohol, the following comparisons are given.

One drink (12 g of alcohol) is equal to:

- 12 ounces of beer,
- 5 ounces of table wine,
- 1.5 ounces of 80 proof liquor,
- 2 to 3 ounces of liquor of aperitif, or
- 8 to 9 ounces of malt liquor.

A drink increases the blood alcohol level in a 150-pound individual by 15 to 20 mg/dL. There is no pattern of alcohol use in adolescents that should be considered acceptable. In adults up to 65 years of age, the threshold of drinking that is, considered risky is 14 or more drinks per week and 4 or more per occasion for adult males, and 7 or more drinks per week and 3 or more per occasion for adult females. However, some universities through the Amethyst Initiative[27] have initiated lowering the drinking age from age 21 to 18. This was met with a lot of resistance, because setting the age limit for alcohol at age 21 was associated with decreased deaths from drunken driving.

Cannabis and K2

Marijuana is the most commonly abused substance among LGBT youth. A common misconception that cannabis is a drug without adverse acute effects and with no long-term consequences contributes to its initiation and continuation. However, there is increasing evidence of adverse effects of chronic marijuana use on human brain development and development of psychosis and mental health problems.[28–30]

Legislative legalization of marijuana is increasingly widespread in the United States. Currently, 23 states and Washington, DC, legalize marijuana for medical use,[31] despite a dearth of scientific evidence supporting the medical use of inhaled marijuana. Diversion is a significant problem, especially among youth. About 74% of the adolescents had used someone else's medical marijuana, with a median of 50 times.[32] The American Psychiatric Association has issued a statement saying that inhaled marijuana is not endorsed for medical purposes.[33] Alaska, Washington, Oregon, and Colorado allow marijuana for recreational purposes.[31]

Recently, there has been an increase in use of a K2 (synthetic marijuana, spice, black mamba, crazy clown). Adverse health effects from K2 have been reported, including severe agitation and confusion, paranoia, hallucinations, and death.[34] This substance poses particularly insidious risks for being abused, including frequent molecular modification by producers that evade both legal regulation and toxicologic screening.

PSYCHIATRIC COMORBIDITY

Many youth with substance abuse problems also have other, cooccurring psychiatric diagnoses ("comorbidity"). For example, the National Comorbidity Survey used a structured diagnostic interview in a representative sample to assess the prevalence and correlates of psychiatric disorders. A subgroup of adolescents, the National Comorbidity Survey—Adolescents (n = 10,000) had a median age of onset of 15 years for substance use. Having a substance use disorder was associated with an increased likelihood of developing a subsequent mood disorder[35] such as major depressive disorder. This underscores the importance of simultaneously addressing all mental health needs in youth with or at risk for substance abuse (see Stewart Adelson and colleagues' article, "Development and Mental Health of LGBT Youth in Pediatric Practice," in this issue).

Substance use is also related to other high-risk behaviors that may increase morbidity and mortality, and place youth's physical health at risk. For example, one study found that LGBT youth reported higher drug use, increased high-risk sexual behaviors, and increased suicidal thoughts or attempts compared with heterosexual youth.[36] Among youth ages 13 to 24 years, young gay and bisexual men accounted for an estimated 19% (8800) of all new HIV infections in the United States, and 72% of new HIV infections among youth in 2010, underscoring the importance of HIV prevention among this group, including addressing any substance abuse.[37]

SUBSTANCE ABUSE PREVENTION

Preventive strategies are already incorporated into general pediatric care settings as part of overall health promotion: health maintenance, nutrition, and sober lifestyle with engagement of the youth and the family in the dialogue during each visit. These can serve to reinforce what may already been offered at school. More focused are training in social skills, communication and assertiveness, anger management, problem-solving skills to more specific areas that are substance focused, and needing referrals (psychoeducation on drug use, its consequences to individual and to the families, refusal skills and like) when abuse is already considered. In some programs, elements are implemented over several years.[38–41] Programs are needed for LGBT youth that address specific risk factors and issues that affect them, and are conducted in a safe and supportive way. However, even in programs not specifically designed for LGBT youth, facilitators can and should be nonjudgmental, caring, empathic and inclusive, consistent with standard mental health practice principles (see Stewart Adelson and colleagues' article, "Development and Mental Health of LGBT Youth in Pediatric Practice," in this issue). Additionally, programs like straight and gay alliances may enhance the inclusion of LGBT youth in general community programs. Structured substance abuse prevention programs are often deployed in schools and other community organizations and agencies. Clinicians should be familiar with programs and resources in their communities and be ready to refer youth at risk or otherwise in need of these.

SCREENING FOR SUBSTANCE ABUSE

As with all health and mental health issues, medical professionals should provide a welcoming and nonjudgmental environment (see Scott E. Hadland and colleagues' article, "Caring for LGBTQ Youth in Inclusive and Affirmative Environments"; and Stewart Adelson and colleagues' article, "Development and Mental Health of LGBT Youth in Pediatric Practice," in this issue) in assessing substance use in LGBT youth.

In addition to resources referenced throughout this volume, standard professional education curricula for medical, nursing and paramedical staff[42–52] include training to help them achieve clinical and cultural competence. Parents of sexual minority youth increasingly look for such providers to meet their child's needs.[53] This approach should be used in eliciting information about drug use as part of routine history taking, in support of a drug-free lifestyle as a part of overall wellness. Few clinic settings provide a full continuum of substance abuse services from screening to active substance abuse treatment. However, screening should be done routinely, and serves to identify those who are abusing substances and in need of treatment, as well as those at risk and possibly benefiting from preventive services.

CLINICAL VIGNETTE: A POSITIVE DRUG USE SCREEN IN A BISEXUAL ADOLESCENT FEMALE

RM is a 14-year-old bisexual female who was referred for a routine physical examination from the local homeless shelter. She recalled being bullied early for her learning and attention difficulties. She was rejected for being "bisexual" forcing her to run away. The assigned physician approached the interview in a nonjudgmental and emphatic manner to make her at ease and to reliably obtain information. She reported that her father was an alcoholic and that she was exposed to domestic violence growing up.

She disclosed twice weekly use of weed and smokes 4 cigarettes daily, started when she ran away from home 2 years ago. She would smoke cigarettes after weed to heighten her high. CRAFFT (Car, Relax, Alone, Forget, Friends, Trouble) was positive at 4. She reported being raped at knifepoint. She is now regular in seeing her therapist and has responded well on fluoxetine.

Along with screening, triaging is necessary to identify any acute safety issues that warrant immediate attention. Examples include intoxications states with changes in mentation or disorientation (cannabis, hallucinogens/psychedelic drugs, inhalants); with prominent agitation/aggression with or without changes in mentation or disorientation (phencyclidine, K2, bath salts); with prominent psychiatric symptoms of hallucinations (cannabis, hallucinogens/psychedelic drugs, phencyclidine); and withdrawal states complicated by suicidal depression (cocaine withdrawal, dextromethorphan).

History from both patients and collateral informants can help the clinician assess the need for further medical intervention, including emergency room evaluation.

As a useful screening tool in some settings, clinicians can consider using an evidenced based screening tool for adolescents known as the "CRAFFT" questionnaire), an acronym for the following 6 questions[54]:

C—Have you ever ridden in a *car* driven by someone (including yourself) who was "high" or has been using alcohol or drugs?

R—Do you use alcohol or drugs to feel *relax*, feel better about yourself, or fit in?

A—Do you ever use alcohol or drugs while *alone* [modified for LGBT youth to: when you feel different or alone]?

F—Do you *forget* things you did while using alcohol or drugs?

F—Do your *family members* and friends ever tell you that you should cut down on your drinking or drug use?

T—Have you gotten into *trouble* while you were using drugs or alcohol?

Although this tool has not been studied in or specifically modified for LGBT youth, it has been reliably used among inpatients[55] and level 1 pediatric trauma settings.[56] A computer version has been found to gather information reliably, and may be a tool to improve office practice efficiency in appropriate settings.[57] Any 2 or more positive response to these questions is indicative of a likely substance use problem[58] in keeping with current *Diagnostic and Statistical Manual of Mental Disorders* (DSM)-5 classification.[59]

Another screening instrument, the Alcohol Use Disorders Identification Test (AUDIT),[60] has been used in randomized controlled trials of adolescent screening, referral and treatment. The domains include alcohol use (frequency and amount), dependence symptoms (loss of control and withdrawal), and harmful consequences. CRAFFT and AUDIT (with a threshold of 8 for responders over the age of 18 and 3 for those younger than 18) have good psychometric predictive values,[58] and are therefore preferable as structured screening instruments with youth, compared with "CAGE"[61] (*Cut down*—Have you ever felt you needed to *cut down* on your drinking? *Annoyed*— Have people *annoyed* you by criticizing your drinking? *Guilty*—Have you ever felt *guilty* about drinking? *Eye-opener*—Have you ever felt you needed a drink first thing in the morning [*eye opener*] to steady your nerves or get rid of a hangover?) with poor specificity and sensitivity in underage drinkers.

These self-report tools have been found to be reliable and valid in majority of adolescents.[62,63] Nevertheless, a subset of adolescents in drug clinics and school settings will deny or minimize their use and collaborative information and objective drug screens can be helpful to support diagnosis and document sobriety.

DIAGNOSIS OF SUBSTANCE ABUSE

In some primary care settings, substance abuse screening will be followed by referral to a mental health or substance use specialist for a full diagnostic evaluation and targeted substance use treatment. In other cases, substance abuse treatment will be integrated with other aspects of pediatric care. Because treatment settings and community resources vary widely, clinicians should plan for the particular needs of LGBT youth, keeping in mind the welcoming health care and mental health principles (see Scott E. Hadland and colleagues' article, "Caring for LGBTQ Youth in Inclusive and Affirmative Environments"; and Stewart Adelson and colleagues' article, "Development and Mental Health of LGBT Youth in Pediatric Practice," in this issue), in familiarizing themselves with available resources and appropriate referral through the continuum of care. The following is an overview of substance abuse evaluation.

The DSM-5 Criteria for Substance use Disorder are given below.

A. Problematic pattern of use leading to clinically significant impairment or distress, manifested by at least 2 of the following:
   1. Often taken in larger amounts or over a longer period than was intended.
   2. Persistent desire or unsuccessful efforts to cut down or control use.
   3. A great deal of time is spent in activities necessary to obtain (drug), use (drug), or recover from its effects.
   4. Craving, or strong desire to use (drug).
   5. Recurrent (drug) use resulting in failure to fulfill major role obligations at work, school, or home.
   6. Continued (drug use) despite having persistent or recurrent social or interpersonal problems caused by the effects of (drug).
   7. Important social, occupational, or recreational activities are given up or reduced because of (drug) use.
   8. Recurrent (drug) use in situations in which it is physically hazardous.
   9. (Drug) use is continued despite knowledge of having a persistent or recurrent physical or psychological problem that is likely to have been caused or exacerbated by (drug).

10. Tolerance to either of the following:
    - A need for markedly increased amounts of alcohol to achieve intoxication or desired effects.
    - Markedly diminished effect with continued use of the same amount of alcohol.
11. Withdrawal, as manifested by either of the following:
    - The characteristic withdrawal syndrome for (drug).
    - (Drug, or a closely related substance), is taken to relieve or avoid withdrawal symptoms.

In addition to the DSM-5 criteria, important aspects of diagnosing substance use involves being mindful of special principles relevant to youth in general and LGBT youth in particular. To assess the problem clearly, it is useful to do a functional assessment of drug use, eliciting a thorough inventory for each drug of abuse on the following:

- Last use, amount, route: to address at the outset the potential for life-threatening withdrawal symptoms (particularly for alcohol, benzodiazepines, and cocaine).
- Onset.
- Context and progression of use; triggers.
- Current amount, frequency (contrasting with past use).
- Positive and negative consequences of drug use.
- Polydrug use (as drugs as commonly used in combination, such as marijuana and nicotine [to boost the high], cocaine and benzodiazepines (drugs that complement each effects to achieve an even high), cocaine and alcohol.
- Periods of sobriety and what supports it.
- Treatment history: of different levels of care (outpatient, intensive outpatient, day program, inpatient detox, rehab, long-term residential halfway houses, etc.); use of medications specific for substance of abuse (to include methadone, buprenorphine, naltrexone, acamprosate, disulfiram); 12 steps, rational recovery, Relapse Prevention; dual diagnosis (substance abuse and psychiatric disorders)

This functional assessment is to establish the presence of substance use disorder using the DSM-5.[64]

CLINICAL VIGNETTE: FUNCTIONAL IMPAIRMENT FROM DRUG USE IN A GAY YOUTH

VA reported smoking weed yesterday, which he started age 13. He was constantly bullied at school because of being gay. In the last year, he started smoking daily to calm him down, because he is more frustrated or angry. Feeling paranoid was infrequent to make him stop. He also enjoys smoking with his peers. Perceived benefits outweigh the risk: "I still get by and [do] not fail." He also started drinking and does not see this as a problem. He refused counseling when seen in the emergency room for alcohol poisoning.

CONFIDENTIALITY

Confidentiality is an important clinical consideration with adolescents, and is particularly so with sexual and gender minority youth (see Scott E. Hadland and colleagues' article, "Caring for LGBTQ Youth in Inclusive and Affirmative Environments"; and Stewart Adelson and colleagues' article, "Development and Mental Health of LGBT Youth in Pediatric Practice," in this issue). Owing to the special issues faced by them in establishing trust in the clinical alliance, issues related to identity disclosure, and possible alienation from peers, family, or other supports, it is important to consider these matters tactfully and to weigh carefully the overall benefits and risks of disclosure in supporting sobriety, safety issues (including adverse physical and medical consequences), and methods of monitoring and involving family, who are often important treatment allies. In many cases, adolescents will agree to share clinical information and treatment with significant others, and family therapy can be an integral part treatment in addition to individual therapy. However, for LGBT youth who are non-disclosed, who are unsure of their identity, or have concerns about adverse family or peer reactions to issues of sexual orientation or gender that cannot be disentangled from substance use issues, the clinician must weigh these factors carefully in the treatment plan, bearing in mind the ethical and legal guidelines regarding privileges of confidentiality. In some cases, it may be useful to obtain expert consultation on these. For patients who have entrenched drug use problems and poor insight or motivation for seeking care, leverage for treatment from external sources, such as protective agencies, Youth Service Bureaus, case managers, or probation may be necessary.

CLINICAL VIGNETTE: THE IMPORTANCE OF CONFIDENTIALITY

Dr M asked GP, a 15-year-old male, how he identifies his sexual preference, during a routine well-child visit. GP disclosed being homosexual. Although he is comfortable about his orientation, he has only "came out" to his close friends and not to his family. GP was assured that this would be kept confidential. He was likewise offered a referral for counseling should he desire to learn how to deal with coming out to his parents. Referral to a substance abuse prevention program was given after GP was found to be at risk for alcohol abuse. This was also made confidentially with clear parameters of defining acute safety issues that would require the pediatrician to disclose alcohol abuse (although not sexual orientation) information to his parents.

TREATMENT OF SUBSTANCE ABUSE

Substance use disorders are best understood as a disease with frequent onset in adolescence, and to be understood in terms of its adverse effects on brain development and its later risk for psychopathology. It negatively impacts skill acquisition and compromises adaptive identity formation. It follows a chronic illness pattern with relapses and remission. The challenge is to move and sustain a level of motivation to change. Drug-using peers negatively impact sobriety and necessitate strengthening of supports by networking with non–drug-using peers.

Level of Care

Substance abuse treatment is ideally undertaken at a level of care commensurate with need. This is laid out in the American Society of Addiction Medicine Patient Placement Criteria 2 Revised (ASAM PPC 2R) levels of care.[65] Treatment is informed by assessing the level of risk in different domains including withdrawal potential, medical complications, comorbid psychiatric conditions, the individual's level of motivation, and their environment. This checklist allows clinicians to assess an individual patient's needs within each of these domains to help determine the least restrictive level of care that is desirable based on the patient's needs (**Table 1**).

Once the level of risk in each domain has been clarified, it can be used in the chart below to determine the level of care desirable for that level of risk, to help clarify the ideal treatment setting. The more severe the risk, the more likely it is that a higher level of care is warranted. Risk may exist simultaneously in several domains; for example, a patient may simultaneously have complicated withdrawal, disorientation, comorbid medical issues like diabetes, psychiatric issues like suicidality, and continuing drug use (**Table 2**). This combination of risks would warrant a heightened level of care, with the most severe risk determining the optimal level.

Table 1 Risk matrix

Dimension	RR-0 None	RR-1 Mild	RR2-Moderate	RR-3 Significant	RR-4 Severe
1. Detox/withdrawal potential					
2. Medical conditions/ complications					
3. Psychiatric					
4. Readiness for change					
5. Relapse/continued use potential					
6. Recovery environment					

AMERICAN SOCIETY OF ADDICTION MEDICINE PATIENT PLACEMENT CRITERIA 2 REVISED

The modified criteria address the need to treat up to 60% of psychiatric disorders cooccurring with substance abuse, the intensity of which differs from minimal to comprehensive. These services are either accessed from without or part of services provided. Adolescents, by virtue of the salient issues they have would usually need a higher level of care when compared with their adult counterparts with the same assigned level.

TREATMENT PRINCIPLES

Substance abuse treatment for youth is best conceived as being embedded within comprehensive services that address the youth as a whole person, considering dimensions of life including family, school, community, and—if appropriate—vocation, treating comorbid psychiatric disorders, addressing safety issues such as violence and suicidality, and threats such as sexually transmitted diseases (HIV, hepatitides, etc).[66] Treatment must be individualized with the use of evidence based treatment, and of sufficient length of time to effect change. Engagement and retention in treatment are paramount.

The following is an overview of evidenced-based substance abuse treatment strategies. This is provided both for those who wish to coordinate care with substance abuse clinicians, and as an information resource for pediatric practitioners who may desire further training in addiction medicine.

EVIDENCE-BASED INTERVENTIONS

Motivational Enhancement Therapy[67] is both an interviewing and a treatment approach that is patient centered. It emphasizes empathy with patients who do not currently see drug use as a problem. The goal is to enhance motivation for behavioral change that will reduce substance abuse by providing the cons over pros of drug use, without the use of argument, direct confrontation or challenges. Therapists "roll with resistance," meeting patients where they currently are in their ability to acknowledge the consequences of substance use with the goal of supporting self-efficacy. This approach emphasizes the adolescent's personal wish to effect change and agency to do so.

Table 2
6 dimensions

Dimensions/Levels of Care	0.5 Early Intervention	I Outpatient	II.1 IOP	II.5 Partial	III.1 Clinically Managed Low Residential III.5 Clinically Managed Medium Intensity III.7 Clinically Managed High-Intensity Residential	IV.7 Medically Monitored Intensive Inpatient	IV Medically Managed Intensive Inpatient	Opioid Maintenance Therapy
1. Detox								
2. Medical								
3. Psychiatric								
4. Readiness for change								
5. Relapse/ continued use potential								
6. Recovery environment								
Dual diagnosis capable								
Dual diagnosis enhanced								

COGNITIVE–BEHAVIORAL THERAPY

Cognitive–behavioral therapy (CBT) is usually provided after a level of motivation to change has been achieved.[68,69] It is important to note that motivation can waver. CBT centers on the following:

- Thinking about the consequences of drug use,
- Self-control and drug-refusal skills,
- Identification and avoidance of high risk situations and problematic behaviors leading to drug use,
- Social networking and prosocial activities,
- Coping with authority and compliance skills,
- Problem solving, and
- Relapse Prevention.

CBT maybe particularly suitable in situations where anxiety and depression are co-morbid, because it can be an effective intervention for these as well.[70–72] An individually tailored Relapse Prevention is then developed.[73]

ADOLESCENT COMMUNITY REINFORCEMENT APPROACH

In this approach, the focus is changing the environment that supports sobriety by:

- Rewarding sober supporting behaviors through the use of vouchers/tokens,
- Withdrawing privileges for drug using behaviors/positive toxicology screens, and
- Behavioral modification of maladaptive behaviors through consequences such as house arrest and/or bracelet monitoring.

This treatment has been demonstrated to be effective in not only decreasing illegal drug use and alcohol, but also decreasing criminal activity, violent behavior, and risky sexual behaviors, as well as improving family functioning.[74,75]

FAMILY THERAPY

Especially in adolescents, this can be a very important component of treatment in:

- Decreasing resistance,
- Addressing substance use as a family problem instead on focusing on the individual alone,
- Interrupting dysfunctional sequences of family behavior,
- Assessing interpersonal function of drug use,
- Implanting change strategies, and
- Teaching assertiveness training in adolescents and at-risk sibling(s).

Effective family functioning, monitoring and supervision, rule setting, parental praise in positive behavior, moderate and consistent discipline, and care and enforcement of family rules serve as models for adaptive behaviors.[76,77] In one study, family therapy is found to have the most effect compared with other therapies though other treatments are effective compared with no treatment at all.[78] For LGBT youth in amenable families, this modality may provide an opportunity to support family acceptance. For those who are nondisclosed, however, the treatment plan needs to take this into account factors like confidentiality, the treatment alliance, and safety appropriately.

TWELVE-STEP PROGRAMS AND OTHER FACILITATION GROUPS

Studies involving the general adolescent population have indicated that, when used, they are more likely to complete treatment and abstain longer. Ways to improve access include promoting such groups as a means to obtain social support, use of "sober schools," teen section in recovery book stores, establishing teen meetings as facilitated by adult mentors within adult meetings or making it a homogenous group of sexual minority youth only.[79–81] Using a workbook, Jaffe[82] has adapted the first 5 steps of Alcoholics Anonymous to suit adolescents by emphasizing power and control. Given the intense group dynamics of 12-step programs, for LGBT youth, it is crucial that these programs be assessed for their ability to provide the individual patient with an appropriately affirming and nonstigmatizing treatment environment. This may require vetting of the program before referral. Information on Alcoholics Anonymous appropriate to youth and access to meetings is available at http://www.aa. org/assets/en_US/f-9_amessagetoteenagers-1.pdf, which provides information in a pamphlet form and includes screening questions on alcohol.

For LGBT youth specifically, special factors that may increase the risk of substance abuse may include exposure to environments like nightclubs that provide opportunities for meeting others and overcoming isolation in which others normalize substance use, or where substances of abuse are available. A subset of youth at risk might use these substances as a maladaptive strategy to relieve shame or other painful affects associated with rejecting interactions and self-stigma. For these youth, substance abuse prevention and treatment may involve providing alternative, adaptive ways of overcoming isolation and shame and achieving pride in their identity without drug use. Treatment that promotes adaptive coping with stigma and support groups, including appropriate 12-steps and other support networks if appropriately nonstigmatizing, welcoming, and inclusive, may be appropriate alternatives for doing so that can decrease the likelihood of substance use.

Medications are used to:

1. Treat comorbid psychiatric disorders such as depression, psychosis or bipolar disorder, and so on;
2. Treat withdrawal effects;
3. As aversive agents (disulfiram);
4. Block reinforcing effects of drugs (naltrexone);
5. Substitute a similar drug for maintenance (methadone, buprenorphine);
6. Substitute a similar drug for taper (nicotine replacements);
7. Reduce craving
8. Reverse life-threatening intoxication (naloxone for opioids, flumazenil for benzodiazepines);
9. As adjuncts (vitamin supplements eg, B_{12}, folate, thiamine for alcohol); and
10. Treat specific drug of abuse, singly or in combination.

Medication studies are very limited to small, double-blind studies and a number are case reports. Applications to adolescents are extrapolated from adults and are used as off label. Medication-assisted therapy is an evidence-based treatment specific for alcohol and opioids, usually combined with psychotherapy to improve efficacy. Disulfiram for alcohol is effective and safe even on a long-term basis.[83] Naltrexone was found to reduce intensity of drinking but not frequency of drinking or heavy drinking days in young adults.[84] Buprenorphine has been used in 15- to 21-year-olds, and when combined with weekly individual and group counseling showed better outcomes when used as maintenance compared with detoxification.[85] Although there are limited studies on methadone for adolescents, they are found to be effective.[86] Medications to treat opioids should be increasingly considered in light of the current opioid epidemic.

Primary practitioners' and pediatricians' comfort level in using medications to treat adolescent psychiatric disorders is influenced by factors including access to training, clinical experience related to practice type and setting, and personal preferences and biases. This is equally true for adolescent substance use disorders. Because psychiatric disorders and substance use are highly comorbid, with the advent of the medical home model with primary care physicians as gatekeepers, it may become increasingly common for primary care practitioners to provide psychopharmacological treatment to youth when needed. In some cases, treatment regimens established by psychiatrists and other mental health specialists will be continued by primary physicians once adolescents have been stabilized and are referred back to them. Consultation with child and adolescent psychiatrists, addiction psychiatrists, pediatricians with an addiction medicine subspecialization, outreach to specialty organizations, and attendance at specific psychopharmacology workshops, are some ways to improve core competencies. Further, certain practice settings in publicly funded programs make it possible for behavioral health services to be incorporated or operate side by side with medical and family practice services. This configuration allows for the coordination of medical, psychiatric, and substance abuse services.

DRUG TESTING

Primary care clinicians may see adolescents referred for drug testing as part of substance abuse or mental health care. Drug testing usually uses urine specimens, although other measures (saliva, blood, hair follicles) are sometimes used. Drug testing may be used as part of a substance abuse treatment plan as an objective means of establishing recovery and as a negative reinforcer in supporting sobriety. **Table 3** gives guidance about half-life and detection time for a variety of substances of abuse, and can be useful in reconciling inconsistencies in the history.[87]

YOUTH SMOKING CESSATION

A recent review showed promise using cognitive–behavioral interventions, although more than 50% of subjects continue to use despite treatment and abstinence rarely persists beyond 3 months.[88] Success is better achieved by discouraging onset of use through public campaign efforts and limiting access. Nicotine Replacement Therapy

Table 3 Half-life and detection time for a variety of substances of abuse		
Drugs	Serum Half-Life (h)	Urine Detection (d)
Amphetamines	10–15	1–2
Barbiturates	20–96	3–14
Benzodiazepines	20–96	3–14
Cocaine	0.8–6	0.2–4
Methaqualone	20–60	7–14
Opiates	2–4	1–2
Phencyclidine	7–16	2–8
Cannabis	10–40	2–8 (acute); 14–42

(NRT) was found to be helpful in achieving abstinence at week 2 in a double blind study.[89] Varenicline was not found associated with increased adverse effects or suicide.[90]

A nicotine vaccine continues to be an area of research that has not yet been clinically applied.[91,92] Group cessation curricula tailored for LGBT populations were found feasible to implement and show evidence of effectiveness. Community interventions have been implemented by and for LGBT communities. Although these interventions showed feasibility, no rigorous outcome evaluations exist.[93] There were very few cessation programs specific for youth. There are data to support that interventions in primary care setting may prevent initiation of smoking.[94] A brief, computer-assisted tobacco intervention counseling increased the rate of smoking cessation.[95]

SUMMARY

Like all youth, a subset of LGBT youth experience substance abuse risk, and some of these will develop substance use problems. LGBT youth have unique developmental experiences and stressors, and preliminary epidemiologic evidence indicates that some of them are at slightly increased risk for these problems in comparison with the general population.

Because LGBT youth are becoming more visible in society, they will require care from pediatricians in established settings and programs within communities, whether school-based programs, in clinics and primary care settings, or in mental health and substance abuse clinics. It is important that their needs be addressed skillfully within these settings. A number of preventive programs, screening, brief interventions, and targeted substance abuse treatments can be applied to LGBT youth. Further research is needed to establish their efficacy for this population and to identify barriers in their implementation for effective programming.

Preventive programs are sometimes available in schools and community settings. A number of these interventions share common themes in fostering skill building, general wellness, and specific refusal skills for youth who are at risk for, but who have not actually developed, substance abuse. A list of these programs (together with a list of treatment clinics) should be readily available as a referral source.

Structured instruments such as CRAFFT and AUDIT can form part of routine screening to be used in wellness programs, along with psychoeducation on drugs, such as information about their adverse effects on the body and brain and their social and educational consequences as well as the benefits of a drug free lifestyle as routine complements to screening.

Effective substance abuse prevention and treatment exists. Incorporating LGBT-specific needs into pediatric substance-abuse related care is a basic clinical competence in pediatrics. Substance abuse screening, assessment, referral and treatment appropriate to LGBT youth should be integrated into routine pediatric practice with the goal of identifying those at elevated risk requiring targeted assessment, referral and treatment.

For LGBT youth with substance abuse, Motivational Enhancement Therapy, alone or in combination with CBT and Relapse Prevention and Family Therapy, can be helpful at different treatment phases. There are limited data on the use of medications in adolescent substance use disorders, with some evidence of their safety and efficacy, especially when combined with targeted psychotherapies. When indicated, medications should be considered. Barriers to use of medications should be addressed, especially if significant psychiatric comorbidity is present. Alcoholic Anonymous has 12-step programs for adolescents, but they may require modification to be specifically appropriate for LGBT youth.

REFERENCES

1. Rosario M, Schrimshaw EW, Hunter J. Different patterns of sexual identity development over time: implications for the psychological adjustment of lesbian, gay, and bisexual youths. J Sex Res 2011;48(1):3–15.
2. Johnston LD, O'Malley PM, Miech RA, et al. Monitoring the Future national survey results on drug use: 1975–2014: Overview, key findings on adolescent drug use. Ann Arbor (MI): Institute for Social Research, The University of Michigan; 2015.
3. Center for Behavioral Health Statistics and Quality. Behavioral health trends in the United States: Results from the 2014 National Survey on Drug Use and Health; 2014. Available at: http://www.samhsa.gov/data/.
4. Centers for Disease Control and Prevention, Youth Risk Behavior Surveillance System (YRBSS). Available at: www.cdc.gov/healthyyouth/yrbs/index.htm.
5. McCabe SE, Hughes TL, Bostwick W, et al. Assessment of difference in dimensions of sexual orientation: implications for substance use research in a college-age population. J Stud Alcohol Drugs 2005;66(5):620–9.
6. Corliss HL, Rosario M, Wypij D, et al. Sexual orientation and drug use in a longitudinal cohort study of U.S. adolescents. Addict Behav 2010;35(5):517–21.
7. Eisenberg ME, Wechsler H. Substance use behaviors among college students with same-sex and opposite-sex experience: results from a national study. Addict Behav 2003;28(5):899–913.
8. Marshal MP, Friedman MS, Stall R, et al. Individual trajectories of substance use in lesbian, gay and bisexual youth and heterosexual youth. Addiction 2009; 104(6):974–81.
9. Wong CF, Kipke MD, Weiss G. Risk factors for alcohol use, frequent use, and binge drinking among young men who have sex with men. Addict Behav 2008; 33(8):1012–20.
10. Garofalo R, Mustanski BS, McKirnan DJ, et al. Methamphetamine and young men who have sex with men: understanding patterns and correlates of use and the association with HIV-related sexual risk. Arch Pediatr Adolesc Med 2007;161(6): 591–6.
11. Li MJ, DiStefano A, Mouttapa M, et al. Bias-motivated bullying and psychosocial problems: implications for HIV risk behaviors among young men who have sex with men. AIDS Care 2014;26(2):246–56.
12. Torres H, Delonga K, Lee S, et al. Socio-contextual factors: moving beyond individual determinants of sexual risk behavior among gay and bisexual adolescent males. J LGBT Youth 2013;10(3).
13. Hightow-Weidman LB, Phillips G 2nd, Jones KC, et al, YMSM of Color SPNS Initiative Study Group. Racial and sexual identity-related maltreatment among minority YMSM: prevalence, perceptions, and the association with emotional distress. AIDS Patient Care STDS 2011;25(Suppl 1):S39–45.
14. Russell ST, Ryan C, Toomey RB, et al. Lesbian, gay, bisexual, and transgender adolescent school victimization: implications for young adult health and adjustment. J Sch Health 2011;81(5):223–30.
15. Huebner DM, Thoma BC, Neilands TB. School victimization and substance use among lesbian, gay, bisexual, and transgender adolescents. Prev Sci 2015; 16(5):734–43.
16. Birkett M, Newcomb ME, Mustanski B. Does it get better? A longitudinal analysis of psychological distress and victimization in lesbian, gay, bisexual, transgender, and questioning youth. J Adolesc Health 2015;56(3): 280–5.

17. Ybarra ML, Mitchell KJ, Palmer NA, et al. Online social support as a buffer against online and offline peer and sexual victimization among U.S. LGBT and non-LGBT youth. Child Abuse Negl 2015;39:123–36.

18. Hawkins JD, Catalano RF, Miller JY. Risk and protective factors for alcohol and other drug problems in adolescence and early adulthood: implications for substance abuse prevention. Psychol Bull 1992;112(1):64–105.

19. Di Chiara G, Bassareo V, Fenu S, et al. Dopamine and drug addiction: the nucleus accumbens shell connection. Neuropharmacology 2004;47(Suppl 1):227–41.

20. Kandel DB, Yamaguchi K, Chen K. Stages of progression in drug involvement from adolescence to adulthood: further evidence for the gateway theory. J Stud Alcohol 1992;53(5):447–57.

21. Huang YY, Kandel DB, Kandel ER, et al. Nicotine primes the effect of cocaine on the induction of LTP in the amygdala. Neuropharmacology 2013;74:126–34.

22. Easton A, Jackson K, Mowery P, et al. Adolescent same-sex and both-sex romantic attractions and relationships: implications for smoking. Am J Public Health 2008;98(3):462–7.

23. Austin SB, Ziyadeh N, Fisher LB, et al. Sexual orientation and tobacco use in a cohort study of US adolescent girls and boys. Arch Pediatr Adolesc Med 2004;158(4):317–22.

24. Tamí-Maury I, Lin MT, Lapham HL, et al. A pilot study to assess tobacco use among sexual minorities in Houston, Texas. Am J Addict 2015;24(5):391–5.

25. Remafedi G, Carol H. Preventing tobacco use among lesbian, gay, bisexual, and transgender youths. Nicotine Tob Res 2005;7(2):249–56.

26. Lamkin L, Davis B, Kamen A. Rationale for tobacco cessation interventions for youth. Prev Med 1998;27(5 Pt 3):A3–8.

27. Amethyst Initiative. Welcome to the Amethyst Initiative. Available at: http://www.theamethystinitiative.org.

28. McQueeny T, DeWitt SJ, Mishra V. Preliminary findings demonstrating latent effects of early adolescent marijuana use onset on cortical architecture. Dev Cogn Neurosci 2015;16:16–22.

29. Bechtold J, Simpson T, White HR, et al. Chronic adolescent marijuana use as a risk factor for physical and mental health problems in young adult men. Psychol Addict Behav 2015;29(3):552–63.

30. Shakoor S, Zavos HM, McGuire P, et al. Psychotic experiences are linked to cannabis use in adolescents in the community because of common underlying environmental risk factors. Psychiatry Res 2015;227(2–3):144–51.

31. Governing. Local government record hiring uptick in July. Available at: www.governing.com/gov-data.

32. Salomonsen-Sautel S, Sakai JT, Thurstone C, et al. Medical marijuana use among adolescents in substance abuse treatment. J Am Acad Child Adolesc Psychiatry 2012 Jul;51(7):694–702.

33. American Psychiatric Association. Position statement on marijuana as medicine. Available at: http://www.psychiatry.org/home/policy-finder.

34. Law R, Schier J, Martin C, et al, Centers for Disease Control and Prevention (CDC). Notes from the field: increase in reported adverse health effects related to synthetic cannabinoid use - United States, January-May 2015. MMWR Morb Mortal Wkly Rep 2015;64(22):618–9.

35. Merikangas KR, He JP, Burstein M, et al. Lifetime prevalence of mental disorders in U.S. adolescents: results from the National Comorbidity Survey Replication–Adolescent Supplement (NCS-A). J Am Acad Child Adolesc Psychiatry 2010;49(10):980–9.

36. Blake SM, Ledsky R, Lehman T, et al. Preventing sexual risk behaviors among gay, lesbian, and bisexual adolescents: the benefits of gay-sensitive HIV instruction in schools. Am J Public Health 2001;91:940–6.
37. Centers for Disease Control and Prevention. HIV Surveillance Report. Available at: http://www.cdc.gov/hiv/library/reports/surveillance/.
38. Gorman DM, Conde E. Conflict of interest in the evaluation and dissemination of "model" school-based drug and violence prevention programs. Eval Program Plann 2007;30(4):422–9.
39. Sanchez RP, Bartel CM. The feasibility and acceptability of "arise": an online substance abuse relapse prevention program. Games Health J 2015;4(2):136–44.
40. Kulis S, Yabiku ST, Marsiglia FF, et al. Differences by gender, ethnicity, and acculturation in the efficacy of the keepin' it REAL model prevention program. J Drug Educ 2007;37(2):123–44.
41. Council on Drug Abuse. Available at: http://www.drugabuse.ca.
42. AAP Committee on Substance Abuse. Substance use screening, brief intervention, and referral to treatment for pediatricians. Pediatrics 2011;128(5):e1330–40.
43. Committee On Adolescence. Office-based care for lesbian, gay, bisexual, transgender, and questioning youth. Pediatrics 2013;132(1):198–203.
44. Moll J, Krieger P, Moreno-Walton L, et al. The prevalence of lesbian, gay, bisexual, and transgender health education and training in emergency medicine residency programs: what do we know? Acad Emerg Med 2014;21(5):608–11.
45. Lapinski J, Sexton P, Baker L. Acceptance of lesbian, gay, bisexual, and transgender patients, attitudes about their treatment, and related medical knowledge among osteopathic medical students. J Am Osteopath Assoc 2014;114(10):788–96.
46. Obedin-Maliver J, Goldsmith ES, Stewart L, et al. Lesbian, gay, bisexual, and transgender-related content in undergraduate medical education. JAMA 2011;306(9):971–7.
47. Lapinski J, Sexton P. Still in the closet: the invisible minority in medical education. BMC Med Educ 2014;14:171.
48. Orel NA. Investigating the needs and concerns of lesbian, gay, bisexual, and transgender older adults: the use of qualitative and quantitative methodology. J Homosex 2014;61(1):53–78.
49. Rutherford K, McIntyre J, Daley A, et al. Development of expertise in mental health service provision for lesbian, gay, bisexual and transgender communities. Med Educ 2012;46(9):903–13.
50. Müller A. Teaching lesbian, gay, bisexual and transgender health in a South African health sciences faculty: addressing the gap. BMC Med Educ 2013;13:174.
51. Callahan EJ, Sitkin N, Ton H, et al. Introducing sexual orientation and gender identity into the electronic health record: one academic health center's experience. Acad Med 2015;90(2):154–60.
52. Dorsen C. An integrative review of nurse attitudes towards lesbian, gay, bisexual, and transgender patients. Can J Nurs Res 2012;44(3):18–43.
53. Shields L, Zappia T, Blackwood D, et al. Lesbian, gay, bisexual, and transgender parents seeking health care for their children: a systematic review of the literature. Worldviews Evid Based Nurs 2012;9(4):200–9.
54. Knight JR, Shrier LA, Bravender MD, et al. A new brief screen for adolescent substance abuse. Arch Pediatr Adolesc Med 1999;153:591–6.
55. Oesterle TS, Hitschfeld MJ, Lineberry TW, et al. CRAFFT as a substance use screening instrument for adolescent psychiatry admissions. J Psychiatr Pract 2015;21(4):259–66.

56. Johnson KN, Raetz A, Harte M, et al. Pediatric trauma patient alcohol screening: a 3 year review of screening at a Level I pediatric trauma center using the CRAFFT tool. J Pediatr Surg 2014;49(2):330–2.

57. Harris SK, Knight JR Jr, Van Hook S, et al. Adolescent substance use screening in primary care: validity of computer self-administered versus clinician-administered screening. Subst Abus 2016;37(1):197–203.

58. Dhalla S, Zumbo BD, Poole G. A review of the psychometric properties of the CRAFFT instrument: 1999-2010. Curr Drug Abuse Rev 2011;4(1):57–64.

59. Mitchell SG, Kelly SM, Gryczynski J, et al. The CRAFFT cut-points and DSM-5 criteria for alcohol and other drugs: a reevaluation and reexamination. Subst Abus 2014;35(4):376–80.

60. Bernstein J, Heeren T, Edward E, et al. A brief motivational interview in a pediatric emergency department, plus 10-day telephone follow-up, increases attempts to quit drinking among youth and young adults who screen positive for problematic drinking. Acad Emerg Med 2010;17:890–902.

61. Ewing JA. Detecting alcoholism: the CAGE questionnaire. JAMA 1984;252(14): 1905–7.

62. Winters KC, Stinchfield RD, Henly GA, et al. Validity of adolescent self-report of alcohol and other drug involvement. Subst Use Misuse 1990;25:1379–95.

63. Winters KC, Kaminer Y. Screening and assessing adolescent substance use disorders in a clinical population. J Am Acad Child Adolesc Psychiatry 2008;47: 740–4.

64. American Psychiatric Association. Diagnostic and statistical manual of mental disorders. 5th edition. Arlington (VA): American Psychiatric Association; 2013.

65. American Society of Addiction Medicine (ASAM). What is the ASAM criteria? Available at: http://www.asam.org/publications/the-asam-criteria/about/.

66. National Institute on Drug Abuse. Principles of adolescent substance use disorder treatment: a research-based guide. Available at: https://www.drugabuse.gov/publications/principles-adolescent-substance-use-disorder-treatment-research-based-guide/principles-adolescent-substance-use-disorder-treatment.

67. Barnett E, Sussman S, Smith C, et al. Motivational interviewing for adolescent substance use: a review of the literature. Addict Behav 2012;37(12):1325–34.

68. Beck A, Weishaar M. Cognitive therapy. In: Corsini RJ, Wedding D, editors. Current psychotherapies. Belmont (CA): Brooks/Cole; 2005.

69. Barrett H, Slesnick N, Brody JL, et al. Treatment outcomes for adolescent substance abuse at 4- and 7-month assessments. J Consult Clin Psychol 2001;69: 802–13.

70. Puleo CM, Conner BT, Benjamin CL, et al. CBT for childhood anxiety and substance use at 7.4-year follow-up: a reassessment controlling for known predictors. J Anxiety Disord 2011;25(5):690–6.

71. Cornelius JR, Douaihy AB, Kirisci L, et al. Longer-term effectiveness of CBT in treatment of comorbid AUD/MDD adolescents. J Med Biol Front 2013;19(2).

72. Esposito-Smythers C, Spirito A, Kahler CW, et al. Treatment of Co-occurring substance abuse and suicidality among adolescents: a randomized trial. J Consult Clin Psychol 2011;79(6):728–39.

73. Larimer ME, Palmer RS, Marlatt GA. Relapse prevention. An overview of Marlatt's cognitive-behavioral model. Alcohol Res Health 1999;23(2):151–60.

74. Curtis SV, Wodarski JS. The East Tennessee assertive adolescent family treatment program: a three-year evaluation. Soc Work Public Health 2015;30(3): 225–35.

75. Godley SH, Smith JE, Passetti L, et al. The Adolescent Community Reinforcement Approach (A-CRA) as a model paradigm for the management of adolescents with substance use disorders and co-occurring psychiatric disorders. Subst Abus 2014;35(4):352–63.

76. Rowe CL. Multidimensional family therapy: addressing co-occurring substance abuse and other problems among adolescents with comprehensive family-based treatment. Child Adolesc Psychiatr Clin N Am 2010;19(3):563–76.

77. Hogue A, Liddle HA. Family-based treatment for adolescent substance abuse: controlled trials and new horizons in services research. J Fam Ther 2009;31(2): 126–54.

78. Tanner-Smith EE, Wilson SJ, Lipsey MW. The comparative effectiveness of outpatient treatment for adolescent substance abuse: a meta-analysis. J Subst Abuse Treat 2013;44(2):145–58.

79. Kelly JF, Brown SA, Abrantes A, et al. Social recovery model: an 8-year investigation of adolescent 12-step group involvement following inpatient treatment. Alcohol Clin Exp Res 2008;32(8):1468–78.

80. Kelly JF, Dow SJ, Yeterian JD, et al. Can 12-step group participation strengthen and extend the benefits of adolescent addiction treatment? A prospective analysis. Drug Alcohol Depend 2010;110(1–2):117–25.

81. Steve Sussman S. A review of alcoholics anonymous/narcotics anonymous programs for teens. Eval Health Prof 2010;33(1):26–55.

82. Jaffe S. Step workbook for adolescent chemical dependency recovery: a guide to the first five steps (5 pack). Washington, DC: American Academy of Child and Adolescent Psychiatry; 1990.

83. Niederhofer H, Staffen W. Comparison of disulfiram and placebo in treatment of alcohol dependence of adolescents. Drug Alcohol Rev 2003 Sep;22(3):295–7.

84. O'Malley SS, Corbin WR, Leeman RF. Reduction of alcohol drinking in young adults by naltrexone: a double-blind, placebo-controlled, randomized clinical trial of efficacy and safety. J Clin Psychiatry 2015;76(2):e207–13.

85. Woody GE, Poole SA, Subramaniam G, et al. Extended vs short-term buprenorphine-naloxone for treatment of opioid-addicted youth: a randomized trial. JAMA 2008;300(17):2003–11.

86. Khuri ET, Millman RB, Hartman N, et al. Clinical issues concerning alcoholic youthful narcotic abusers. Adv Alcohol Subst Abuse 1984;3(4):69–86.

87. Bukstein OG, Bernet W, Arnold V, et al. Practice parameter for the assessment and treatment of children and adolescents with substance use disorders. J Am Acad Child Adolesc Psychiatry 2005;44:6.

88. Simon P, Kong G, Cavallo DA, et al. Update of adolescent smoking cessation interventions: 2009-2014. Curr Addict Rep 2015;2(1):15–23, 80.

89. Scherphof CS, van den Eijnden RJ, Engels RC, et al. Short-term efficacy of nicotine replacement therapy for smoking cessation in adolescents: a randomized controlled trial. J Subst Abuse Treat 2014;46(2):120–7.

90. Molero Y, Lichtenstein P, Zetterqvist J, et al. Varenicline and risk of psychiatric conditions, suicidal behaviour, criminal offending, and transport accidents and offences: population based cohort study. BMJ 2015;350:h2388.

91. Hoogsteder PH, Kotz D, van Spiegel PI, et al. Efficacy of the nicotine vaccine 3'-AmNic-rEPA (NicVAX) co-administered with varenicline and counselling for smoking cessation: a randomized placebo-controlled trial. Addiction 2014; 109(8):1252–9.

92. Cornish KE, de Villiers SH, Pravetoni M, et al. Immunogenicity of individual vaccine components in a bivalent nicotine vaccine differ according to vaccine formulation and administration conditions. PLoS One 2013;8(12):e82557.
93. Lee JG, Matthews AK, McCullen CA, et al. Promotion of tobacco use cessation for lesbian, gay, bisexual, and transgender people: a systematic review. Am J Prev Med 2014;47(6):823–31.
94. Patnode CD, O'Connor E, Whitlock EP, et al. Primary care-relevant interventions for tobacco use prevention and cessation in children and adolescents: a systematic evidence review for the U.S. Preventive Services Task Force. Ann Intern Med 2013;158(4):253–60.
95. Hollis JF, Polen MR, Whitlock EP, et al. Teen reach: outcomes from a randomized, controlled trial of a tobacco reduction program for teens seen in primary medical care. Pediatrics 2005;115(4):981–9.

Body Image and Eating Disorders Among Lesbian, Gay, Bisexual, and Transgender Youth

Zachary McClain, MD*, Rebecka Peebles, MD

KEYWORDS

- Adolescents • LGBT youth • Eating disorders • Body image • Mental health
- Gender identity

KEY POINTS

- Current studies suggest that sexual minority males have increased body shape and weight dissatisfaction, anorexic and bulimic symptoms, and may consider physical appearance to be critical to their sense of self.
- Studies have shown that transgender youth and young adults report elevated rates of compensatory behaviors (eg, vomiting, laxative use, or diet pill use) and higher rates of past-year self-reported eating disorders.
- Transgender adults may be at increased risk for eating disorders, so screening and early recognition of disordered eating are critical in youth.
- Although further research is needed to examine the relationships among disordered eating, gender identity, and sexual orientation, current literature suggests that sexual minority youth of both genders may be more likely to engage in dangerous weight control behaviors.

INTRODUCTION

Adolescence is a crucial period for emerging sexual orientation and gender identity, and body image disturbance and disordered eating. Eating disorders are serious mental illnesses with the potential for life-threatening medical complications and death.[1–3] Although previously body image distortion and disordered eating were considered to affect only a small subset of society, largely affluent females, they are now recognized to impact millions, including all individuals along the sexual orientation and gender identity spectrum.[3,4] However, most research on eating disorders

---

Disclosure Statement: The authors have nothing to disclose.
Craig Dalsimer Division of Adolescent Medicine, The Children's Hospital of Philadelphia, 34th Street and Civic Center Boulevard, 11 Northwest Tower, Room 10, Philadelphia, PA 19104, USA
* Corresponding author.
E-mail address: mcclainz@email.chop.edu

Pediatr Clin N Am 63 (2016) 1079–1090
http://dx.doi.org/10.1016/j.pcl.2016.07.008
pediatric.theclinics.com

and body image has focused on heterosexual, cisgender individuals.[5] The limited amount of research on sexual minority adolescents and gender variant youth suggests associations between sexual orientation and gender identity and eating-related pathology.[6] Eating disorders in youth have recently been shown to be highly associated with the future development of serious psychiatric conditions, such as anxiety disorders, depression, drug use, and self-harm behaviors in young adulthood.[7] It is of paramount importance that health care providers recognize the importance of eating and body image issues and that these may affect the lesbian, gay, bisexual, transgender (LGBT) population in unique ways, and may confer future risk toward adverse health outcomes. An American Academy of Pediatrics' statement in the office-based care for LGBT youth has called for additional research in this area, highlighting eating disorders as an underresearched, critical, and emerging issue for LGBT youth.

OVERVIEW OF EATING DISORDERS AND BODY IMAGE

Eating disorders are common and potentially deadly conditions. They affect millions of males and females in the United States, with some estimates up to 30 million Americans, with increasing incidence and prevalence, and with adolescents diagnosed with increasing frequency.[8,9] The precise cause of these disorders is not known. It is most likely that they are multifactorial in origin, with evidence for neurobiologic predispositions and gene-environment interactions.[10,11] Among the wide spectrum of mental illness, eating disorders have the highest rate of mortality, making them a considerable public health concern.[12–14] These facts are particularly important for LGBT adolescents who are at elevated risk for certain other psychiatric comorbidities. Therefore, it is of critical importance that providers are aware of how to detect these disorders in LGBT youth.

Previously, eating disorders were divided into three major subgroups: (1) anorexia nervosa (AN), (2) bulimia nervosa (BN), and (3) eating disorder not otherwise specified. However, the *Diagnostic and Statistical Manual of Mental Disorders, 5th Edition* (DSM-5) has broadened the diagnostic criteria in a more inclusive manner to reduce the need for eating disorder not otherwise specified.[15] Other diagnoses described in the DSM-5 include: pica, rumination disorder, avoidant/restrictive food intake disorder (ARFID), binge-eating disorder, other specified feeding or eating disorder, and unspecified feeding or eating disorder.[16] Estimates show that AN affects up to 1% of adolescents and young adults, whereas BN has a prevalence of 3%.[14,17,18] Although some individuals may not meet the full criteria for an eating disorder diagnosis, many adolescents engage in eating disordered behaviors, with up to 25% of high school aged girls and 11% of high school aged boys reporting disordered eating severe enough to need evaluation, and 9% of high school girls and 4% of boys reporting daily vomiting to control their weight.

In contrast to eating disorders, body image is less strictly defined and less extensively studied. Body image can loosely be defined as how individuals perceive themselves when they picture themselves in their minds or see themselves in the mirror. Body image includes how one feels about not only their body, but also their height, weight, and shape. This article looks at disturbances or distortions in body image, often described as body dissatisfaction.

It is important to notice that the DSM-5 allows not only distortions in how body weight or shape are experienced as a feature defining eating disorders diagnostically, but also allows behaviors that sabotage weight gain as a criterion. This is important, because many pediatric and adolescent patients do not report body image disturbances as part of their eating disorder, and are less able to identify cognitive changes brought on by their disease.

Finally, it is critical to note that for the most part, most sexual minority youth have positive body image and lack eating concerns. This article discusses associations found in the literature between sexual minority youth and eating disorders or body image disturbances.

CLINICAL PRESENTATION, SCREENING, AND TREATMENT

A patient with weight loss, inability to gain weight, restrictive thoughts about weight or shape, unexplained vomiting, or abnormal behaviors around eating warrants a consideration of the diagnosis of an eating disorder. AN typically presents with a refusal to maintain a minimally normal body weight, or behaviors that consistently sabotage weight gain even in the absence of overt cognitions surrounding weight and/or shape. Pediatric patients may present with failure to gain weight over time as normally expected, and sometimes with linear growth stunting, rather than weight loss. BN typically presents as recurrent episodes of binge eating followed by compensatory behaviors to avoid weight gain, such as laxative use, induced vomiting, fasting, or purging with exercise.[19] Finally, ARFID is another common disorder that presents with nonorganic, often anxiety-mediated causes of poor growth and feeding resulting in impairments in physical health, growth, and/or psychosocial functioning. Patients with ARFID do not have concerns about their weight or shape that can be identified, but nonetheless have difficulty eating adequately.

Some presentations of eating disorders, however, are less obvious, and include chronic abdominal pain, syncope, orthostatic hypotension, chest pain, menstrual irregularities or other symptoms of hypogonadism, and constipation. Eating disorders are not always clear on initial presentation and a high index of suspicion is warranted if these signs are present. In fact, patients with dangerous eating disorders may be overweight or obese, and may therefore not be recognized. Similarly, eating disorders are often missed in adolescent and young adult males at first presentation, and it is important to consider these diseases when males present with symptoms that may reflect an eating disorder.

When assessing a patient with a suspected eating disorder, the provider must first determine the patient's current weight, examine a weight and growth history, and compare the current weight with an expected body weight or body mass index (BMI). A comprehensive history and physical examination should be completed. Caregivers and patients should be interviewed, because some adolescents and young adults with eating disorders can significantly underreport their symptoms. In addition to common history questions, questions about diet, body image, weight-control measures, and psychiatric conditions should be assessed. Suggested screening questions are listed in **Box 1**.[20]

Box 1
Some suggested screening questions for an eating disorder

Have you done anything in the past 6 months to change your weight?

What do you think you ought to weigh?

How much do you exercise?

How do you feel if you miss a workout?

What is your self-image (thin or fat)?

Are there any particular areas of your body that bother you?

The diagnosis of an eating disorder is a clinical diagnosis and there is not confirmatory laboratory testing. However, some laboratory and ancillary testing may be helpful in the evaluation of a patient with an eating disorder (**Box 2**). The purpose of such testing is to exclude other organic etiologies, detect complications of malnutrition or vomiting, and initially assess the effects of nutritional rehabilitation.

Once an eating disorder has been suspected or diagnosed by a provider, depending on their comfort level, they may want to refer patients for further evaluation and management. Eating disorders are complex and are ideally treated by an experienced multidisciplinary team of medical, nutrition, and mental health professionals. Many inpatient facilities that treat patients with eating disorders use specific protocols. Inpatient treatment is appropriate for patients who are medically unstable (eg, because of bradycardia, hypotension, hypothermia, electrolyte abnormalities, arrhythmias) or psychiatrically unstable (concurrent suicidality, severe self-injury, or other dangerousness to self or others), or for patients who cannot otherwise be treated in a home setting.[3,20,21]

Although family acceptance is a special issue for LGBT youth (See Sabra Katz-Wise and colleagues article, "LGBT Youth and Family Acceptance," in this issue), when feasible, treatment paradigms have shifted away from individualized therapy for most adolescents and young adults, to family-based therapy. Family-based therapy is an outpatient intervention with a multidisciplinary team that places parental involvement at the center of care and is critical to the therapeutic success of the adolescent. When feasible, family-based therapy is currently the gold standard and is the most effective treatment of AN and BN.[22] Individual treatment paradigms on general populations are less successful in randomized trials. If family members cannot be leveraged to help support the adolescent, thought should be given to involving other caretakers or adults in treatment, because it seems that full recovery is much more challenging when done without a strong support system.

PRACTICAL TIPS IN MANAGING EATING DISORDERS

Treatment paradigms have shifted dramatically. This is caused by improved understanding that eating disorders can be conceptualized as brain disorders that respond

---

Box 2
Laboratory screening when considering an eating disorder

Complete blood count

Erythrocyte sedimentation rate or C-reactive protein

Comprehensive metabolic panel, phosphorus, magnesium

Thyroid studies

Celiac panel

25-OH Vitamin D

Ferritin, iron studies

Thiamine, B_{12} levels

Estradiol or testosterone

Follicle-stimulating hormone and luteinizing hormone

Prolactin

Pregnancy testing

If liver function elevated, consider Wilson disease, porphyria

best to weight restoration and normalization of eating behaviors. These disorders are now widely accepted to have strong genetic links in families, and occur in young people with genetic and neurobiologic vulnerability. Family members are critical to supporting a patient in recovery.[21]

It is helpful when treating a patient with an eating disorder to focus on reversing maladaptive eating behaviors that have developed and restoring weight, rather than diverting time and effort to speculation about causation that cannot be substantiated. Although a risk factor, sexual orientation or gender identity concerns are clearly neither necessary nor sufficient to cause eating disorder, because most sexual minority or transgender youth never develop an eating disorder. If they do, this is likely influenced by the same genetic and neurobiologic vulnerabilities as in nonsexual and gender minority peers.

Weight restoration to a goal that is consistent with the patient's prior, premorbid growth trajectories earlier in childhood is important. Obviously, not all patients are meant to live at the fiftieth percentile for BMI. Some may need to be higher or lower, consistent with their premorbid BMI.

Because eating disorders can be chronic and are associated with significant morbidity and mortality, providers should discuss their concerns with patients and families early and refer to experienced teams for treatment. Evidence-based treatment that involves families should be prioritized if available and feasible. These illnesses should be recognized as treatable, and full recovery should be the goal, because they do not need to be chronic.[3,20,21] **Box 3** provides treatment recommendations.

SEXUAL ORIENTATION AND EATING DISORDERS AND BODY IMAGE

Eating disorders or disordered eating behaviors peak during the psychosocial developmental period of adolescence.[13] Adolescence is also a critical developmental

---

Box 3
Practical treatment tips for youth with eating disorders

1. Have a high index of suspicion. These are common illnesses in adolescence.

2. Make the diagnosis and have the discussion with your patient and his/her family. Do not be afraid of upsetting the family, and do not wait for a large medical work-up to be complete before discussing openly that an eating disorder is a likely cause of your patient's symptoms. This conversation can be initiated while completing the necessary medical work-up, rather than after. This will help your patient feel more supported early on.

3. Instill hope. These disorders can be fully treated, and full recovery should be the goal.

4. Impress an appropriate sense of medical urgency. Treatment should not be delayed, and will not get easier in time. These are life-threatening illnesses if they go untreated.

5. Target behaviors. If weight gain needs to occur, that should be the initial focus. If other behaviors are more important, such as purging, work with a team of professionals to target those.

6. Set accurate weight goals that align with your patient's prior growth history. Not everyone is meant to weigh less than the fiftieth percentile.

7. Refer to qualified providers with demonstrated track records of success for treatment. This is more important than providers who are close to home or have convenient schedules. Just as with any other serious illness, the quality and background of the treating specialist is important to reach success.

8. Support the family. Patients should not be treated in isolation. Embrace the involvement of family members or friends if they are able to be structured and supportive in targeting the treatment goals. These illnesses are best fought with caregivers who can help.

period for sexual orientation. Given the proximity of emergence of eating disorders and sexual orientation during this critical developmental stage, it is not surprising that eating disorders may disproportionately affect vulnerable youth, particularly sexual minority youth.[23]

For many years, the literature has described relationships between disordered eating, body image dissatisfaction, and sexual orientation in adults. Early studies showed that up to 42% of men diagnosed with an eating disorder have identified as homosexual or bisexual.[24–26] Community-based studies have shown that homosexual men may be more vulnerable to eating disorders and have greater body dissatisfaction and increased bulimic and anorexic symptoms compared with heterosexual men.[24,27,28] Additionally, early studies that surveyed men who identify as homosexual have demonstrated that they have increased body shape and weight dissatisfaction than heterosexual men.[29–31] These same studies also showed that homosexual men consider physical appearance to be critical to their sense of self.

Only a few studies have explored associations between sexual orientation and eating disorders in adolescents. Early school-based studies have shown that gay boys and boys with same-sex partners had more disordered eating behaviors and more body dissatisfaction when responding to a health behavior survey.[32,33] In a large longitudinal sample of Norwegian high school students, girls and boys with same-sex sexual experience at entry were three and seven times more likely to report bulimic behaviors 5 years later. Same-sex attraction in boys at entry had higher odds for bulimic symptoms compared with heterosexual boys, even when adjusting for other posited risk factors for bulimia.[34]

A longitudinal cohort study of adolescent boys and girls living in the United States examined eating behaviors across the sexual orientation spectrum. In this community-based study, they constructed a sexual orientation scale that was based on the participants' described feelings of sexual attraction. The scale varied from completely heterosexual to completely homosexual. Other categories of sexual orientation included mostly heterosexual, bisexual, mostly homosexual, and unsure. "Mostly heterosexual" adolescents, who are distinct from "completely heterosexual" adolescents, comprised a significant portion of the cohort. Boys and girls in this group indicated more weight and appearance concerns than their same-gender heterosexual counterparts. Additionally, "mostly heterosexual" girls had higher rates of dieting and eating-disordered behaviors than their heterosexual counterparts.[35] In contrast, the same study found that lesbian and bisexual girls were happier with their bodies, put less effort to look like those in the media, and did less dieting than their heterosexual counterparts. Alternatively, gay and bisexual boys put more effort to look like those in the media and had increase bingeing compared with their heterosexual counterparts.

This study was expanded to look at sexual orientation–related differences in purging and binge eating and found that those adolescents who identified as lesbian, gay, and bisexual (LGB), showed higher past-year prevalence of binge eating and purging compared with heterosexuals.[23] Data from the Youth Risk Behavioral System Survey in 2005 and 2007 confirmed many of these associations longitudinally, showing that LGB high school boys and girls were significantly more likely to develop purging and diet pill use.[36]

A population-based sample of high school students examining associations between health risk behaviors and sexual orientation found sexual minority youth participating in unhealthy weight control practices. Overall, they found a higher prevalence of students reporting same-sex sexual behaviors were more likely to engage in unhealthy weight control practices than those reporting opposite-sex sexual behaviors.

Additionally, this study found that students reporting both-sex sexual behaviors were significantly more likely to engage in vomiting and using laxatives to lose weight or to keep from gaining weight in the preceding 30 days.[37]

Finally, another large study of college students showed that lesbian and bisexual women were more likely than their heterosexual counterparts to engage in unhealthy weight control behaviors; these same associations were not shown in sexual minority college men.[38] In another study, LGB college men showed significantly higher odds of reporting both clinical eating disorders and disordered eating behaviors when compared with heterosexual men; both LGB men and women were significantly more likely to report dieting to lose weight compared with their heterosexual peers.[39]

Similar associations have been noted in a prospective cohort study of youth that investigated issues including the development of body image concerns, the Growing Up Today Study. Although not a random sample of US adolescents, and with few youth of color, this study is key in addressing sexual orientation disparities in vulnerability to eating disorder symptoms. In this study, although heterosexual boys were also at risk of body image concerns, sexual minority boys had a higher likelihood of developing body image concerns and weight-control behaviors associated with wanting to be lean as they grew older.[40] Sexual minority youth were more likely to show disparities between their actual and perceived weight statuses, with gay and bisexual boys more likely to perceive themselves as overweight when they were in a normal weight category, and lesbian girls more likely to perceive themselves as normal weight when they were actually overweight or obese. Sexual minority youth of both genders were also significantly more likely to engage in dangerous weight control behaviors.[41] Gay college men have also shown a higher incidence of drive for thinness, body dissatisfaction, and body image–related anxiety than their heterosexual counterparts. These relationships were also more likely to be mediated by media exposure in gay male college students than their heterosexual peers.[42]

Moving beyond community-based studies and looking at clinical samples of adolescents diagnosed with an eating disorder, similar trends are found. It has been reported that nearly 5% to 7% of American adolescents identify as LGBT.[43,44] A study looking at eating behaviors and health in adolescents diagnosed with an eating disorder found a higher prevalence of minority sexual orientation at 8.8%.[45] Furthermore, and in line with previous research in adults and community-based studies in adolescents, this study found that adolescent boys were more likely to endorse minority sexual orientation than adolescent girls. Although previous studies have demonstrated links between disordered eating behaviors and minority sexual orientation in adolescent boys, this study is the first study to examine these associations in adolescents with a clinical diagnosis of an eating disorder.

GENDER IDENTITY AND EATING DISORDERS AND BODY IMAGE

It is evident from the research presented that most studies on disordered eating and body image have centered on cisgender, as opposed to transgender, individuals. Primarily, the research on gender and eating disorders and body dissatisfaction examines the relationship between gender roles (ie, masculinity and femininity) and disordered eating.[46–48] However, no larger studies have examined these associations in youth.

A recent review revealed 26 studies that examine gender identity and disordered eating and body dissatisfaction; however, only one study in the review explored why transgender individuals may be at risk for eating disorders. In general, this review posited that the risk of eating disorders may be secondary to the distress that transgender individuals experience as part of their body dissatisfaction.[49] The review also identified a study that found that male-to-female transgender individuals engage in disordered eating.[50] No literature to date have definitively determined the role of gender identity in the cause of these disorders in transgender or other populations; more research is clearly needed. Thus, it is best for clinicians to focus on effective treatment.

Looking more closely at these studies, transgender adults qualitatively reported themes of disordered eating and drive for thinness as suppressing features of biologic gender and also for some, supporting aspects of desired gender. Some eating disorder behaviors were reported as relieved by gender reassignment.[51] The few case reports available in adolescent and adult transgender patients reveal similar themes of body dissatisfaction and disordered eating, and the authors suggest considering desired gender in developing the treatment strategy for transgender youth patients with eating disorders.[52–57] When looking at the gender identity spectrum, one study showed that individuals that had "conflicted gender identity" demonstrated more symptoms and concerns characteristic of eating disorders on a standardized self-report measure.[58]

A study examining data from the American College Health Association's National College Health Assessment (consisting of 289,024 students from 223 US universities) looked at gender identity and eating disordered behaviors. They found that transgender individuals reported elevated rates of compensatory behaviors (eg, vomiting, laxative use, or diet pill use) in the past 30 days. Additionally, they found that transgender students and cisgender sexual minority male students had higher rates of past-year self-reported eating disorder diagnosis compared with their cisgender heterosexual female counterparts.[5] There is much research needed to better understand the relationships between gender identity, body image, and eating disorders.

WEIGHT REGULATION AND OBESITY

Obesity is not an eating disorder; it is simply a descriptive term indicating a weight status, similar to underweight. The Institute of Medicine notes that there are a few studies indicating that female sexual minority youth and bisexual youth of both genders may be more likely to be obese than their peers.[36,59] Sexual minority males seem to be at reduced risk of BMI gains from year to year in adolescence.[36,60]

Weight status becomes a medical concern if it risks adversely impacting growth, development, physical health, and or psychosocial functioning. It is important to evaluate weight status in the context of a youth's general health. If someone is underweight compared with other family members without medical reason, this is likely to impact their future growth and pubertal status, and should be worked up medically and addressed nutritionally. However, if another adolescent is also underweight, but so is his or her entire family, or he/she was a product of a premature delivery and has always been small proportionately, then this is likely less of an issue; simply being somewhat underweight may or may not be problematic for an individual adolescent. The same principle can be applied to overweight adolescents. If someone is overweight, but is able to exercise regularly, enjoys a healthy social life, eats a wide variety of nonprocessed foods, and has no metabolic disruptions, then his or her weight status is of less medical concern than if they have obstructive sleep apnea and type II diabetes, and are gaining weight yearly and doing fewer activities because they feel embarrassed, which likely deserves work-up and intervention.

Treatment of obesity commonly involves lifestyle interventions surrounding nutrition and exercise, and has a low success rate in reducing BMI; many therefore promote behavior change for improved quality of life and metabolic health rather than for reducing weight.[61] Treatment should focus on common sense interventions that reduce stigma and target adolescents who are at risk of impairment in one or more health domains, rather than simply treating a number on a scale. More research is needed before any conclusions are drawn about screening or treatment of obesity specifically in sexual and gender minority groups.

SUMMARY

Eating disorders are conditions associated with significant morbidity and mortality that peak during the adolescence period. Eating disorders affect individuals along the sexual orientation and gender identity spectrum. The extant literature suggests that LGBT youth are particularly vulnerable to eating disorders and body dissatisfaction. Because of this, medical providers should screen for disordered eating in LGBT youth, and should know that effective treatments are available. In particular, sexual minority males have greater body dissatisfaction, and more frequently report unhealthy weight control practices, disordered eating behaviors, and classic eating disorders. Additionally, transgender individuals are at risk of eating disorders. Furthermore, disordered eating in LGBT and gender variant youth may be associated with poorer quality of life and mental health outcomes. Obesity may occur more frequently in sexual minority females. More research is needed to determine whether there are specific interventions or targets for sexual minority youth that may be most effective; for now, treatment should focus on therapies that have empiric support in generalized youth populations. As providers, it is important to be aware that these illnesses occur more frequently in LGBT youth and can be fully treated. For these reasons, providers should carefully assess any eating or body image struggles their patients may be experiencing.

REFERENCES

1. Herzog DB, Greenwood DN, Dorer DJ, et al. Mortality in eating disorders: a descriptive study. Int J Eat Disord 2000;28(1):20–6.
2. Katzman DK. Medical complications in adolescents with anorexia nervosa: a review of the literature. Int J Eat Disord 2005;37(Suppl):S52–9 [discussion: S87–9].
3. Rosen DS. Identification and management of eating disorders in children and adolescents. Pediatrics 2010;126(6):1240–53.
4. Peebles R, Lysrter-Mensh LC, Kreipe R. Eating disorders. In: Ginsburg K, Kinsman S, editors. Reaching teens: wisdom from adolescent medicine. Elk Grove Village (IL): American Academy of Pediatrics; 2013. p. 413–23.
5. Diemer EW, Grant JD, Munn-Chernoff MA, et al. Gender identity, sexual orientation, and eating-related pathology in a national sample of college students. J Adolesc Health 2015;57(2):144–9.
6. Coker TR, Austin SB, Schuster MA. The health and health care of lesbian, gay, and bisexual adolescents. Annu Rev Public Health 2010;31:457–77.
7. Micali N, Solmi F, Horton NJ, et al. Adolescent eating disorders predict psychiatric, high-risk behaviors and weight outcomes in young adulthood. J Am Acad Child Adolesc Psychiatry 2015;54(8):652–9.e1.
8. Golden NH, Katzman DK, Kreipe RE, et al. Eating disorders in adolescents: position paper of the Society for Adolescent Medicine. J Adolesc Health 2003;33(6):496–503.

9. Wade TD, Keski-Rahkonen A, Hudson J. Epidemiology of eating disorders. In: Tohen M, editor. Textbook in psychiatric epidemiology. New York: Wiley; 2011. p. 343–60.

10. Mazzeo SE, Bulik CM. Environmental and genetic risk factors for eating disorders: what the clinician needs to know. Child Adolesc Psychiatr Clin N Am 2009;18(1):67–82.

11. Hudson JI, Mangweth B, Pope HG Jr, et al. Family study of affective spectrum disorder. Arch Gen Psychiatry 2003;60(2):170–7.

12. Sullivan PF. Mortality in anorexia nervosa. Am J Psychiatry 1995;152(7):1073–4.

13. Hudson JI, Hiripi E, Pope HG Jr, et al. The prevalence and correlates of eating disorders in the National Comorbidity Survey Replication. Biol Psychiatry 2007; 61(3):348–58.

14. Swanson SA, Crow SJ, Le Grange D, et al. Prevalence and correlates of eating disorders in adolescents. Results from the national comorbidity survey replication adolescent supplement. Arch Gen Psychiatry 2011;68(7):714–23.

15. Call C, Walsh BT, Attia E. From DSM-IV to DSM-5: changes to eating disorder diagnoses. Curr Opin Psychiatry 2013;26(6):532–6.

16. American Psychiatric Association, American Psychiatric Association. DSM-5 Task Force. Diagnostic and statistical manual of mental disorders DSM-5. Arlington (VA): American Psychiatric Association,; 2013. 1 electronic text.

17. Sigel E. Eating disorders. Adolesc Med State Art Rev 2008;19(3):547–72, xi.

18. Hoste RR, Labuschagne Z, Le Grange D. Adolescent bulimia nervosa. Curr Psychiatry Rep 2012;14(4):391–7.

19. Klein DA, Walsh BT. Eating disorders: clinical features and pathophysiology. Physiol Behav 2004;81(2):359–74.

20. Rome ES, Ammerman S, Rosen DS, et al. Children and adolescents with eating disorders: the state of the art. Pediatrics 2003;111(1):e98–108.

21. Campbell K, Peebles R. Eating disorders in children and adolescents: state of the art review. Pediatrics 2014;134(3):582–92.

22. Lock J, Le Grange D, Agras WS, et al. Randomized clinical trial comparing family-based treatment with adolescent-focused individual therapy for adolescents with anorexia nervosa. Arch Gen Psychiatry 2010;67(10):1025–32.

23. Austin SB, Ziyadeh NJ, Corliss HL, et al. Sexual orientation disparities in purging and binge eating from early to late adolescence. J Adolesc Health 2009;45(3): 238–45.

24. Carlat DJ, Camargo CA Jr, Herzog DB. Eating disorders in males: a report on 135 patients. Am J Psychiatry 1997;154(8):1127–32.

25. Herzog DB, Norman DK, Gordon C, et al. Sexual conflict and eating disorders in 27 males. Am J Psychiatry 1984;141(8):989–90.

26. Olivardia R, Pope HG Jr, Mangweth B, et al. Eating disorders in college men. Am J Psychiatry 1995;152(9):1279–85.

27. Russell CJ, Keel PK. Homosexuality as a specific risk factor for eating disorders in men. Int J Eat Disord 2002;31(3):300–6.

28. Carlat DJ, Camargo CA Jr. Review of bulimia nervosa in males. Am J Psychiatry 1991;148(7):831–43.

29. Yager J, Kurtzman F, Landsverk J, et al. Behaviors and attitudes related to eating disorders in homosexual male college students. Am J Psychiatry 1988;145(4): 495–7.

30. Herzog DB, Newman KL, Warshaw M. Body image dissatisfaction in homosexual and heterosexual males. J Nerv Ment Dis 1991;179(6):356–9.

31. Silberstein LR, Mishkind ME, Striegel-Moore RH, et al. Men and their bodies: a comparison of homosexual and heterosexual men. Psychosom Med 1989; 51(3):337–46.

32. French SA, Story M, Remafedi G, et al. Sexual orientation and prevalence of body dissatisfaction and eating disordered behaviors: a population-based study of adolescents. Int J Eat Disord 1996;19(2):119–26.

33. Ackard DM, Fedio G, Neumark-Sztainer D, et al. Factors associated with disordered eating among sexually active adolescent males: gender and number of sexual partners. Psychosom Med 2008;70(2):232–8.

34. Wichstrom L. Sexual orientation as a risk factor for bulimic symptoms. Int J Eat Disord 2006;39(6):448–53.

35. Austin SB, Ziyadeh N, Kahn JA, et al. Sexual orientation, weight concerns, and eating-disordered behaviors in adolescent girls and boys. J Am Acad Child Adolesc Psychiatry 2004;43(9):1115–23.

36. Austin SB, Nelson LA, Birkett MA, et al. Eating disorder symptoms and obesity at the intersections of gender, ethnicity, and sexual orientation in US high school students. Am J Public Health 2013;103(2):e16–22.

37. Robin L, Brener ND, Donahue SF, et al. Associations between health risk behaviors and opposite-, same-, and both-sex sexual partners in representative samples of Vermont and Massachusetts high school students. Arch Pediatr Adolesc Med 2002;156(4):349–55.

38. Laska MN, VanKim NA, Erickson DJ, et al. Disparities in weight and weight behaviors by sexual orientation in college students. Am J Public Health 2015; 105(1):111–21.

39. Matthews-Ewald MR, Zullig KJ, Ward RM. Sexual orientation and disordered eating behaviors among self-identified male and female college students. Eat Behav 2014;15(3):441–4.

40. Calzo JP, Masyn KE, Corliss HL, et al. Patterns of body image concerns and disordered weight- and shape-related behaviors in heterosexual and sexual minority adolescent males. Dev Psychol 2015;51(9):1216–25.

41. Hadland SE, Austin SB, Goodenow CS, et al. Weight misperception and unhealthy weight control behaviors among sexual minorities in the general adolescent population. J Adolesc Health 2014;54(3):296–303.

42. Carper TL, Negy C, Tantleff-Dunn S. Relations among media influence, body image, eating concerns, and sexual orientation in men: a preliminary investigation. Body Image 2010;7(4):301–9.

43. Chandra A, Mosher WD, Copen C, et al. Sexual behavior, sexual attraction, and sexual identity in the United States: data from the 2006-2008 National Survey of Family Growth. Natl Health Stat Report 2011;(36):1–36.

44. Gates GJ. Demographics and LGBT health. J Health Soc Behav 2013;54(1):72–4.

45. McClain Z, Sieke E, Cheek C, et al. Gender differences in minority sexual orientation and quality of life among adolescents with eating disorders in Pediatric Academic Societies. Washington, DC: 2013.

46. Blashill AJ. Gender roles, eating pathology, and body dissatisfaction in men: a meta-analysis. Body Image 2011;8(1):1–11.

47. Murnen SK, Smolak L. Femininity, masculinity, and disordered eating: a meta-analytic review. Int J Eat Disord 1997;22(3):231–42.

48. Williamson I. Why are gay men a high risk group for eating disturbance? European eating disorders review. New York: John Wiley & Sons; 1999.

49. Jones BA, Haycraft E, Murjan S, et al. Body dissatisfaction and disordered eating in trans people: a systematic review of the literature. Int Rev Psychiatry 2016; 28(1):81–94.
50. Khoosal D, Langham C, Palmer B, et al. Features of eating disorder among male-to-female transsexuals. Sex Relation Ther 2009;24:217–29.
51. Algars M, Alanko K, Santtila P, et al. Disordered eating and gender identity disorder: a qualitative study. Eat Disord 2012;20(4):300–11.
52. Ewan LA, Middleman AB, Feldmann J. Treatment of anorexia nervosa in the context of transsexuality: a case report. Int J Eat Disord 2014;47(1):112–5.
53. Murray SB, Boon E, Touyz SW. Diverging eating psychopathology in transgendered eating disorder patients: a report of two cases. Eat Disord 2013;21(1):70–4.
54. Strandjord SE, Ng H, Rome ES. Effects of treating gender dysphoria and anorexia nervosa in a transgender adolescent: lessons learned. Int J Eat Disord 2015; 48(7):942–5.
55. Surgenor LJ, Fear JL. Eating disorder in a transgendered patient: a case report. Int J Eat Disord 1998;24(4):449–52.
56. Turan S, Poyraz CA, Duran A. Prolonged anorexia nervosa associated with female-to-male gender dysphoria: a case report. Eat Behav 2015;18:54–6.
57. Hepp U, Milos G. Gender identity disorder and eating disorders. Int J Eat Disord 2002;32(4):473–8.
58. Ålgars M, Santtila P, Sandnabba NK. Conflicted gender identity, body dissatisfaction, and disordered eating in adult men and women. Sex Roles 2010;63(1–2): 118–25.
59. Institute of Medicine. The health of lesbian, gay, bisexual, and transgender people: building a foundation for better understanding. Washington, DC: The National Academies Press; 2011.
60. Katz-Wise SL, Blood EA, Milliren CE, et al. Sexual orientation disparities in BMI among U.S. adolescents and young adults in three race/ethnicity groups. J Obes 2014;2014:537242.
61. Peebles R. Adolescent obesity: etiology, office evaluation, and treatment. Adolesc Med State Art Rev 2008;19(3):380–405, vii.

The Intersection of Sociocultural Factors and Health-Related Behavior in Lesbian, Gay, Bisexual, and Transgender Youth
Experiences Among Young Black Gay Males as an Example

Errol Fields, MD, PhD, MPH[a], Anthony Morgan, AAS[b],
Renata Arrington Sanders, MD, MPH, ScM[c],*

KEYWORDS

- LGBT • Youth • Gay • Young black gay and bisexual men • YBGBM
- Health-related behavior • Intersectionality • Black/African American

KEY POINTS

- Young black gay and bisexual men (YBGBM) experience multiple inequities compared with their majority peers by virtue of their membership in multiple oppressed and marginalized groups.
- Intersectionality suggests that multiple social identities intersect at the individual or micro level of experience and reflects larger social–structural inequities experienced on the macro level.
- Intersecting identities predispose YBGBM to adverse health outcomes and health inequality, which are further modified by promoting and protective factors.

R.A. Sanders disclosed that she was funded by NICHD K23 HD074470 award.
[a] Division of General Pediatrics and Adolescent Medicine, Johns Hopkins School of Medicine, 200 North Wolfe Street, Baltimore, MD 21287, USA; [b] Division of General Pediatrics and Adolescent Medicine, Johns Hopkins School of Medicine, 200 North Wolfe Street, Baltimore, MD 21287, USA; [c] Division of General Pediatrics and Adolescent Medicine, Johns Hopkins School of Medicine, 200 North Wolfe Street, Baltimore, MD 21287, USA
* Corresponding author.
E-mail address: rarring3@jhmi.edu

BACKGROUND

Intersectionality is a theoretic framework that suggests that multiple social identities—for example, race, ethnicity, gender, and sexual orientation—intersect at the individual or micro level of experience and reflects larger social–structural inequities experienced on the macro level.[1,2] This article uses an intersectionality framework to describe how multiple stigmatized social identities can create unique challenges for young black gay and bisexual men (YBGBM) as an example.

Adolescence is an important time of physical, social, emotional, and cognitive growth and development in the life course.[3] The majority of sexual minority (eg, lesbian, gay, bisexual, and transgender [LGBT]) youth of color emerge from this period as healthy adults, having successfully achieved these developmental tasks.[3] However, relative to their majority peers, these youth face greater, formidable risks to their health and development.[4,5] YBGBM and other young black men who have sex with men (YBMSM), in particular, carry one of the greatest public health burdens in the United States, disproportionately accounting for more than one-half (55%) of all new HIV infections in young men who have sex with men.[6] YBGBM experience multiple inequities compared with their majority peers by virtue of their membership in multiple oppressed and marginalized groups.

There is limited health-focused research on the intersecting identities of young black gay, bisexual, and other men who have sex with men[1,7] but using the lens of intersectionality to understand the threats to health and well-being these young men face may provide key opportunities for prevention and intervention. In this article, we examine the key intersecting identities such as race, sexual identity, and cultural expectations (eg, masculinity, and religious morality; **Fig. 1**) that exist for YBGBM and how such factors may predispose young men to adverse health outcomes and health inequality. We also describe sociocontextual promoting and protective factors that may further

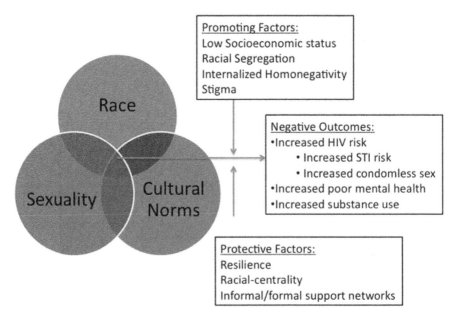

Fig. 1. Key intersecting identities of young black gay and bisexual men. HIV, human immunodeficiency virus; STI, sexually transmitted infection.

modify this relationship, as well as clinical pearls that practitioners can use to help mitigate risk and negative outcomes in YBGBM. Although this article predominantly focuses on HIV risk in YBGBM, many of the key concepts described in this article, such as intersectionality, can be applied to the lived experiences of all LGBT youth that occupy multiple identities.

RACIAL AND SEXUAL IDENTITIES

One of the key tasks of adolescence is identity development,[8] a stage where adolescents and emerging adults come to understand the specific ways in which they fit into society. This task involves developing one's self-concept, which includes both personal identity or perception of self[8] and group identities—that is, membership and identification with a group of people with shared characteristics salient to an individual's self-concept.[9] Racial or ethnic identity, for example, is a group identity based on common heritage and a common sense of identity, affecting one's internal self-concept and interactions with others.[10] Racial/ethnic identity is oftentimes more significant to the self-concept among ethnic minorities and racially oppressed groups.[11] Several theorists have argued that racial identity may be more salient for blacks relative to whites overall because of specific discrimination and racial prejudice blacks have historically faced in the United States[12] and the shared struggle for equity and acceptance within the majority population.[11,12]

Sexual identity development in YBGBM, as in other LGBT youth, involves 2 related processes: identity formation (awareness, questioning and exploration of sexuality) and identity integration (incorporation of sexuality into one's self-concept). Identity integration has been further conceptualized as involvement in lesbian-, gay-, or bisexual- (LGB) related social activities, resolving homonegative attitudes, becoming comfortable with others knowing about an LGB sexual identity, and disclosing sexual identity to important others.[13] Identity formation and integration of developmental processes are often nonlinear and variable across and within individuals. This variability is normal, but difficult or delayed identity integration has been associated with poor markers of psychosocial adjustment in youth including depression and anxiety, conduct problems, and poor self-esteem.[13]

Disclosing sexual identity or "coming out" is not uniformly adaptive; rather, the benefit of coming out depends on social context.[14] Norm compliance and collectivism rather than individualism and self-expression in racial/ethnic minority groups may be more important in the process of sexual identity development in sexual minorities of color than uniform disclosure seen in other groups.[15] For example, Legate and colleagues[14] (2011) found that coming out was associated with higher self-esteem and less depression and anger in autonomy-supportive contexts (ie, interpersonal support for authentic self-expression) but not in controlling social contexts (ie, interpersonal pressure to conform to sociobehavioral norms). As such, affiliation with sexual minority communities and LGB-related social events has been described as less relevant for YBGBM.[16]

Additionally, YBGBM may experience a conflict between same-sex sexuality and homonegative (ie, heterosexist, antigay) cultural expectations of masculinity and religious morality.[17,18] Because of this conflict, some YBGBM may experience or fear that they will experience rejection, ridicule, and isolation from family, peers, and community during key moments in adolescent development. For a group that often identifies first with their racial identity,[19,20] and draws strength and support from that community,[21] preserving that connection may be paramount to "coming out" or otherwise embracing or assuming a gay/bisexual identity.[18,22] Rather than risking that connection, an individual, whose dominant identity is his racial identity, may compartmentalize his sexual identity.[18] In this context, nondisclosure of sexuality may be protective and adaptive by allowing the individual to preserve important social supports.[23] However, as sexual and racial minority youth, the internal conflict some young men wage between cultural expectations and their sexuality may further isolate them at a time when interpersonal attachments are important,[24] particularly if this conflict precludes them from accessing other, appropriate sources of social support related to their sexuality.[25]

CULTURAL NORMS AND EXPECTATIONS
Masculinity

Normative and dominant masculinity in American culture has been described as antifeminine, homophobic, heterosexist, and misogynistic.[26] Some have suggested that stereotypical male gender roles of hypermasculinity (ie, exaggeration of traditional masculine roles through behaviors such as sexual prowess, physical dominance, aggression, competition, and antifemininity) seen in some black men may be a way for black men disempowered by a social context of limited access to socioeconomic power, racism, and discrimination by a predominantly white male society to demonstrate power and authority[22,27] and to approximate the American masculine ideal.

This compensatory expression of hypermasculinity has been suggested as an important coping strategy for racism, oppression, and marginalization, particularly in young black men. Majors' and Billson's[27] conceptual framework "Cool Pose," describes a hypermasculine strategy embraced by black males to cope with and survive in the face of social oppression and racism. Lacking the resources to obtain the traditional American societal prescription for masculinity, "Cool Pose" fosters the development of compulsive masculinity as an alternative to traditional definitions of manhood that "compensates for feelings of shame, powerlessness and frustration" by typifying toughness, sexual promiscuity, and violence to resolve personal conflicts.[27]

The expression of hypermasculinity among black men has also been associated with community and peer acceptance as well as fortification of self-image and self-esteem.[28] In contrast with the expression of hypermasculinity, disclosure of homosexuality has been associated with depressive distress, alienation, and social isolation within black communities.[29] These social sanctions are due, in part, to perceived direct contradictions between "hypermasculine" gender role expectations for black men and association of homosexuality with exaggerated stereotypes of being weak and effeminate.[30,31] YBGBM may alter their presentation or expression of masculinity as a strategy to either avoid ridicule or to fit in and maintain social ties with important others.[32,33]

Although maximizing social reward and avoiding social sanctions are strong motivators, achieving or striving for these homonegative masculine expectations carries significant risk for YBMSM. Fields and colleagues[32] (2015) applied gender role strain theory to a sample of YBMSM who felt pressured to conform to homonegative expectations of masculinity from important others—for example, family, peers, and community. In this analysis, they found examples of psychosocial distress, efforts to camouflage or hide same-sex behavior and identity, strategies to prove one's masculinity, and the potential for increased HIV risk through social isolation, poor self-esteem, reduced access to HIV prevention messages, and limited parental involvement in the development and exploration of sexuality. Moreover, the norm of nondisclosure of same-sex behavior in black communities where homosexuality is viewed as incompatible with masculine expectations[18,26,32] can create opportunities for HIV risk for YBGBM, including exploration of sexuality in hidden, high-risk, often age-discordant, settings such as from the Internet and telephone-based venues.

Religion

Religiosity and religious affiliation have generally been associated with positive mental and physical health outcomes in both cross-sectional and prospective studies.[34,35] However, among sexual minorities, the beneficial impact of religion is less clear. Religious affiliation, although protective in some ways, has also been associated with mental health pathology in YBGBM including psychological distress, depression, poor self-esteem, and internalized homophobia.[36] This relationship between religious affiliation and internalized homophobia has been described by minority stress theory, which posits that health disparities affecting sexual minorities are the result of differential exposure to stigma, homophobia, and rejection[37] (see Mark L. Hatzenbuehler and John E. Pachankis' article, "Stigma and Minority Stress as Social Determinants of Health Among LGBT Youth: Research Evidence and Clinical Implications," in this issue). As a result of this process, some LGBT youth may disassociate more from institutional religion as a coping strategy to avoid the stressors associated with homonegative and potentially stigmatizing social environments.[38]

The salience of religiosity in black communities may limit the value and relevance of disassociation as a coping strategy for YBGBM. The Black Church, a term that refers to the 7 historically black protestant denominations founded after the Free African Society of 1787 and representing more than 80% of black Christians in the United States,[39] is a central religious, social, and cultural institution in black American society. It is uniformly recognized as the most influential institution in black American society[39] and has been at the center of social and political activity throughout history, leading the Civil Rights movement, and other social justice issues related to racial oppression and discrimination.[40] The Black Church has also been a refuge from discrimination and marginalization for black communities.[40] Upwards of 80% report religion as an important part of their lives,[41] and for many of these individuals religion and affiliation with the Black Church as a religious and sociocultural institution are salient to both their self-concept and their black identity.[42,43]

Although black churches are not a monolithic entity and do not uniformly object to homosexuality, many, like other religious institutions, do espouse proscriptive messages against same-sex behavior and identities.[40] The Black Church as an institution has generally been described as homophobic and intolerant of same-sex sexuality[40] and is one of the principal sources of homonegative messages in black communities,[31,33,40] influencing churchgoers and nonchurchgoers alike. In some churches, this message is manifested as silence during the AIDS crisis[40] and in others, the message manifests as explicit and consistent condemnation of homosexuality and homosexual persons.[30,33] This is sometimes replicated in families, among peers, and in the larger community. In addition to the morality of homosexuality, the conflation of gender and sexuality in masculine socialization as described is also entwined in the homonegative messages,[31] which further emasculates such men by making them incapable of meeting expectations for men in the church or in the larger community.[31,44,45]

YBGBM are challenged with significant conflict at the intersection of their same-sex behavior and sexual identity, racial identity, and religiosity. For many, the church environment is highly salient to other aspects of their multiple and intersecting identities and central to black American life and black racial identity.[43] In studies of YBGBM experiences with religiosity, many describe managing this conflict by compartmentalizing their sexual identity within religious contexts. Balaji and colleagues[33] (2012) in a qualitative study of 16 YBMSM (19–24 years of age) described study participants engaging in 'role-flexing,' a strategy for maintaining masculine expectations and camouflaging or concealing sexual orientation to avoid exposure to direct homonegative prejudice in religious settings. This strategy may place youth, particularly those who have not integrated their sexual identity into their sense of self (ie, identity integration), at risk for internalizing many of the homonegative messages they seek to avoid.[30,33] Others, often older adults, described managing this conflict by integrating their religiosity and sexuality through attending religious institutions (often nonblack or non-Christian) that affirmed same-sex sexuality, creating new religious communities outside of traditional church environments, abandoning institutional religion in favor of a more personal and individual relationship with a higher power, or remaining in traditional black religious institutions and rejecting homonegative or nonaffirming messages.[46,47]

Promoting Factors

In the preceding sections, we provided a conceptual approach to understanding how intersecting identities like race, gender, and culture impact one's risk for adverse health outcomes. Marginalization for YBGBM can be promoted further by factors like poverty and low socioeconomic status, racial segregation, homonegativity, stigma, and limited social connectedness. YBGBM, for example, are often disproportionately burdened by the socioeconomic inequity and poor social and built environment that increases risk for HIV and other poor outcomes relative to their white sexual minority peers.[48] **Table 1** reviews these promoting factors further and summarizes how these factors increase risk for HIV and other health and social disparities for YBGBM. Factors such as poverty, social environment (including racial segregation), homonegativity, stigma, and limited social connectedness can further isolate YBGBM predisposing them for risk. Such factors further perpetuate macrolevel factors that impact on the individual level.

Protective Factors

Despite the prevalence of stigma, discrimination, and marginalization, most YBGBM are remarkably resilient, develop coping strategies, build social support networks, and have good mental health.[85] YBGBM often have access to several protective factors despite the challenges they face as sexual and racial/ethnic minorities. Aspects of their dual, intersecting identities that may create adversity (strong ties to racial/ethnic communities, religious or spiritual faith) also tend to be sources of strength. **Table 2** reviews racial centrality, resilience, religiosity and spirituality, and social support, and how these factors can be protective in the lives of YBGBM. These factors can sometimes buffer the negative effect of existing within multiple marginalized identities. For example, prior work suggests that for some YBGBM a positive societal view of black men was associated with decreased sexual risk behavior.[87]

Clinical Considerations

YBGBM are a unique population existing at the intersection of 4 often medically underserved groups, that is, male, young, black, and sexual minority. Additionally, many often are from economically depressed settings. Each of these groups has historically had poor relationships with health care settings. Males are less likely to access primary care, health promotion, or preventive services compared with female patients.[92] Youth have similar barriers; a normal component of adolescent development is the illusion of invulnerability and invincibility; however, this illusion has been correlated with risk behaviors and poor engagement in health care and health promotion.[93] Black individuals have characteristically had low levels of health care use as a result of historical and contemporary barriers to care, including financial and structural access barriers, medical mistrust, and history of unequal and maltreatment.[94] Sexual minorities have similarly had barriers to care resulting from poor cultural competency and low provider knowledge of the health care needs of gay, lesbian, bisexual, and transgender individuals.[95] Although disparities in HIV may have increased access to HIV testing and other preventive health services in underserved areas, those in economically depressed areas have significant barriers to care including cost and insurance,[96] transportation,[97] and competing socioeconomic needs (eg, employment, food, housing).

YBGBM at the intersection of all of these social categories face all of these challenges. Moreover, these challenges are not simply additive; rather, they are interdependent and mutually reinforcing.[1,2] Very few studies have explored the health care experiences of YBGBM. Although some have focused on primary care or preventive health services the majority focus on engagement and retention of HIV-infected youth. Reflecting the multiple challenges discussed, these studies have found the following factors were positively associated with treatment engagement, retention and health care use: feeling respected in clinical settings, receipt of social services ethnic identity affirmation, and employment,[77] whereas negative self-image, medical mistrust, racial and sexual orientation stigma from providers, and stigma disclosing same-sex behavior were negatively associated.[77] In a qualitative study, adult black MSM described experiences of racial and sexual discrimination in medical settings that compounded similar experiences in other aspects of their lives and negatively impacted their medical use, HIV testing, communication with providers, and medication and treatment adherence.[98]

SUMMARY AND RECOMMENDATIONS

We have used an intersectionality framework to describe how occupying multiple stigmatized social identities can create unique challenges for YBGBM as an example. Such intersection can predispose YBGBM to risk and poor health outcomes. Young black gay, bisexual, and other men who have sex with men must achieve the tasks of adolescence at the intersection of multiple social categories such as race, socioeconomic status, gender (and gender expression), religion, and sexuality. This experience is compounded by multiple threats to their health and well-being from their social environment at the interpersonal, intermediate structural, and macrostructural levels. These threats reflect the social inequities this group is disproportionately burdened with as members of multiple oppressed and marginalized groups.

When caring for YBGBM, it is important bear in mind the importance of culture, family and religion in identity development and to assess the following: (1) the social context in which the adolescent lives in (to assess contextual factors that may predispose some YBGBM to risk), (2) a youth's identities, including racial, sexual and cultural group identity, (3) to whom youth have disclosed their sexual orientation, and (4) whether they must exist in certain environments (hypermasculine, religious, etc) that prohibit them from disclosing their sexual orientation to others.

Clinicians should also keep in mind that promoting factors (eg, racial segregation, homonegativity, and stigma) could modify exposure to risk to increase poor outcomes, whereas protective factors (eg, resilience, race centrality, and social support) may help to protect YBGBM from risk. Although this article focused primarily on YBGBM, the intersectionality framework discussed here is also an important lens for other LGBT youth of color and other racial/ethnic groups who may have to cope

Table 1
Promoting factors affecting adverse health outcomes among YBGBM

Domain	Key Points
SES and the structural, social and built environment	• Racial disparities in health can be explained by differences in SES and low SES has been associated with health-related behaviors and poor health outcomes.[49,50] Structural, social, and the built environment (where people live) also explains many of these disparities.[51] HIV and other poor outcomes are often clustered in areas stricken by poverty, crime, high density of alcohol outlets, poorly performing schools, food deserts, vacant houses, and other markers of underinvestment in infrastructure and social services.[52] • These areas are often characterized by socioeconomic inequity, which can lead to negative health outcomes through poor social cohesion, low collective efficacy, and physical and social disorder.[53] • Several studies have demonstrated an association between the social and environmental context of disadvantaged neighborhoods and sexual risk behavior or sexual outcomes among heterosexual adolescents and emerging adults.[53] Far fewer studies of this sort have been done among YBMSM; however, there is evidence of similar associations. In a study of 1289 YBMSM (18–29), socioeconomic distress (as measured by less than a high school degree or GED, less than full-time employment, annual income of less than $20,000, in the past year borrowing money to meet basic needs or running out of money at least once, ever being incarcerated, and ever being homeless) was associated with CAI, a significant risk factor for HIV.[54] A similar study of 328 Detroit YMSM (age 18–29), demonstrated those with income below the poverty line were less likely to have ever been tested for HIV and more likely to report CAI with a serodiscordant partner. In the same study, YMSM living in neighborhoods with greater socioeconomic disadvantage were more likely to have had an HIV test and less likely to report CAI with serodiscordant partners, a finding authors postulate may be due to targeted HIV control efforts to address HIV disparities in underserved areas.[55]
Racial segregation of sexual networks and HIV risk	• New HIV infections among YBMSM (aged 13–24) continue to outpace other racial/ethnic MSM subgroups in the United States,[6] despite equivalent or lower rates of individual HIV risk behavior.[56] • Racial/ethnic segregation—particularly in poor, urban, inner-city environments—has left black and other racial/ethnic minorities disproportionately affected by both low SES and social and built environments that negatively impact health.[57] Public health surveillance data and several studies have demonstrated that black MSM are more likely to live in neighborhoods with lower income[58,59] and higher HIV prevalence[58,59] and are more likely to have lower individual SES compared with white MSM.[58] • Evidence suggests that HIV disparities affecting YBMSM are perpetuated by differences in their sexual networks, including greater race concordance and age discordance between sex partners, higher sexual density (ie, extent to which members are having sex with each other), and greater likelihood of residence in neighborhoods with high HIV prevalence in YBMSM sexual networks.[48,60–63] • Another notable difference is the racial segregation of sexual networks. Preference for black partners has been described in qualitative studies of young and adult black MSM[17,18,64] and likely reflects salience of black identity and desire for shared experiences.[65,66] However, there is also evidence of marginalization of blacks in sexual minority communities that contributes to the racial homogeneity of the sexual networks of black MSM.[67,68]

IH	• IH is an unconscious process where negative societal messages about lesbian, gay, bisexual people become internalized by lesbian, gay, and bisexual persons.[37]
	• The impact of IH on health outcomes has been unclear, but strongest associations have been seen with mental health outcomes, where higher IH predicts greater internalizing mental health problems (eg, depression and anxiety).[69] There have also been positive associations reported between IH and guilt, shame, and low self-esteem and evidence that IH also predicts poor sexual identity development and nondisclosure of sexual identity.[70]
	• Youth-specific studies have been limited, but existing work has demonstrated links between IH and unsafe sexual behaviors, substance use, and nondisclosure of sexual orientation among sexual minority youth.[69,70]
	• Internalized homophobia has also been shown to vary by race and class with greater IH associated with black race, lower education, poverty, homelessness, and history of incarceration.[71] Qualitative studies of YBGBM and adult black MSM have consistently described internalization of homonegative messages among study participants, the negative impact on psychological well-being, and the mechanism by which these ill effects can lead to increased HIV risk.[29,72]
Stigma	• Black gay and bisexual men experience stigma and discrimination in the form of isolation and detachment from both the black and the gay communities.[73,74]
	• The personal experience of stigma, homophobia, and discrimination related to one's race and sexual orientation has been directly related sexual risk behavior including condom nonuse[54], poorer mental health outcomes, including low self-esteem, increased depression, anxiety, suicidal ideation and suicide attempts[37,75], and maladaptive coping strategies, including substance abuse and engaging in fewer health-seeking behaviors.[76]
	• HIV-related stigma additionally impacts care for HIV-infected and at-risk YBGBM and has been associated with a delay in care seeking after HIV diagnosis and nonadherence to HIV medical appointments[77] and may be a barrier to HIV and other sexual health promotion screening services.[78]
	• Minority stress theory suggest that it is the additive effect of socially based membership in marginalized groups that further magnifies the type of social stress that is the result of one's environment.[79]
Limited social connections	• YBGBM are less likely, compared with their white peers, to benefit from connectedness to sexual minority communities. The experience of racism in predominantly white sexual minority communities has been cited as a deterrent to seeking connectedness or support from these communities.[67,80]
	• Black gay, bisexual, and other MSM often describe social isolation and lack of social support from black communities and, in qualitative studies, have consistently reported the absence of organized communities and opportunities to connect with and support one another, citing homophobia and secrecy around same-sex behaviors as contributing factors.[72]
	• Instead, opportunities for interpersonal and peer social interaction, particularly for young men, have been limited to pornography,[81] sexual venues, and social media outlets.[7,82] This social isolation and lack of social support can have deleterious effects on identity development, self-mastery, and self-esteem,[83] lead to IH and identity concealment[29] and contribute to sexual and other risk behaviors.[84]

Abbreviations: CAI, condomless anal intercourse; HIV, human immunodeficiency virus; IH, internalized homonegativity; MSM, men who have sex with men; SES, socioeconomic status; YBGBM, young black gay and bisexual men; YBMSM, young black men who have sex with men.

Table 2
Protective factors affecting the health of YBGBM

Domain	Key Points for Primary Care Providers
Race centrality	• Racial centrality, the degree to which racial identity is central to one's overall identity, has been consistently identified as a protective factor against negative health-related outcomes in African American/black adolescents.[86] • Prior work suggests for some YBGBM high racial centrality and racial public regard (beliefs about how society views black people) was associated with decreased sexual risk behavior including CAI.[87]
Resilience	• YBGBM may be more resilient than their heterosexual and nonminority peers because they occupy 2 identities that have been historically stigmatized in American society.[1] • Studies suggest young black gay/bisexual and other MSM have substantial resilience operationalized through their inner strength, positive social relationships, altruism and the ability to create communities and sources of support.[72] • Researchers have suggested that some protective resilience occurs as a result of the high returns and connectedness of being a part of a racial/ethnic identity and may be in excess, and thus, protective of the returns experienced as part of sexual minority communities.[16]
Religiosity and spirituality	• There is evidence that religiosity and spirituality can also be protective among YBGBM. Prior work of racially diverse YBMSM suggests faithfulness and frequent formal religious attendance was associated with less CAI with male partners.[88] • Other work suggests YBGBM experience psychological benefit from church attendance and religious affiliation despite any homonegative messages present in this social environment.[46] Even among those who have left traditional church affiliations, spirituality remains a salient component of their self-concept and source of strength and resilience.[47]
Social support	• Parental and family support provides resources to cope with social adversity and predicts positive well-being and health outcomes[14] including reduced depression and increased self-esteem[89] for racial and sexual minority youths. • For youth rejected by their families, seeking support from sexual minority communities can be an important and effective coping strategy. Community connectedness seems to be protective against homonegativity and homophobia and has been associated with psychological well-being in YBGBM.[90] • In some urban settings there are community-based organizations developed by and for black sexual minority communities (eg, Gay Men of African Descent in New York City),[16] and several studies have described informal communities and gay 'family' structures in and outside of the House and Ball Culture[91] where sexual minority youth of color are provided social support from older peers that act as parental figures when parental support is absent.

Abbreviations: CAI, condomless anal intercourse; MSM, men who have sex with men; YBGBM, young black gay and bisexual men; YBMSM, young black men who have sex with men.

with specific sociocultural factors related to sexual orientation, gender expression or gender identity that influence health outcomes. Clinicians should be aware of the unique challenges that impact sexual and gender minority groups that occupy multiple marginalized circles to adequately assess, develop programs and cultivate skills in YBGBM that promote protective factors and block the impact of negative promoting factors.

REFERENCES

1. Bowleg L. "Once you've blended the cake, you can't take the parts back to the main ingredients": Black gay and bisexual men's descriptions and experiences of intersectionality. Sex Roles 2013;68(11–12):754–67.

2. Collins PH. Black feminist thought: knowledge, consciousness, and the politics of empowerment. New York: Routledge; 1991.

3. Levine DA, Committee on Adolescence. Office-based care for lesbian, gay, bisexual, transgender, and questioning youth. Pediatrics 2013;132(1):e297–313.

4. Bruce D, Harper GW. Operating without a safety net: gay male adolescents and emerging adults' experiences of marginalization and migration, and implications for theory of syndemic production of health disparities. Health Educ Behav 2011; 38(4):367–78.

5. Collier KL, van Beusekom G, Bos HM, et al. Sexual orientation and gender identity/expression related peer victimization in adolescence: A systematic review of associated psychosocial and health outcomes. J Sex Res 2013;50(3–4):299–317.

6. Centers for Disease Control Prevention. Estimated HIV incidence in the United States, 2007-2010. HIV Surveillance Supplemental Report. 2012 17(4). Available at: http://www.cdc.gov/hiv/topics/ surveillance/resources/reports/#supplemental. Accessed August 18, 2016.

7. Jamil OB, Harper GW, Fernandez MI. Sexual and ethnic identity development among gay–bisexual–questioning (GBQ) male ethnic minority adolescents. Cultur Divers Ethnic Minor Psychol 2009;15(3):203.

8. Erikson EH. Growth and crises of the "healthy personality". In: Erikson EH, Senn MJE, editors. Symposium on the healthy personality. Oxford (England): Josiah Macy Jr. Foundation; 1950. p. 91–146.

9. Tajfel H. Social identity and intergroup relations. European studies in social psychology. Cambridge (United Kingdom): Cambridge University Press; 1982. p. 528. Editions de la Maison des sciences de l'homme. xv.

10. Helms JE. Introduction: review of racial identity terminology. In: Helms JE, editor. Black and White racial identity: theory, research, and practice. Westport (CT): Praeger; 1990. p. 3–8.

11. Phinney JS. Ethnic identity exploration in emerging adulthood. In: Browning DL, editor. Adolescent identities: a collection of readings. New York: The Analytic Press/Taylor & Francis Group; 2008. p. 47–66.

12. Phinney JS. When we talk about American Ethnic Groups, what do we mean? Am Psychol 1996;51:918–27.

13. Rosario M, Schrimshaw EW, Hunter J. Different patterns of sexual identity development over time: implications for the psychological adjustment of lesbian, gay, and bisexual youths. J Sex Res 2011;48(1):3–15.

14. Legate N, Ryan RM, Weinstein N. Is coming out always a "good thing"? Exploring the relations of autonomy support, outness, and wellness for lesbian, gay, and bisexual individuals. Soc Psychol Personal Sci 2012;3(2):145–52.

15. Constantine MG, Gainor KA, Ahluwalia MK, et al. Independent and interdependent self-construals, individualism, collectivism, and harmony control in African Americans. J Black Psychol 2003;29(1):87–101.

16. Moradi B, Wiseman MC, DeBlaere C, et al. LGB of color and White individuals' perceptions of heterosexist stigma, internalized homophobia, and outness: comparisons of levels and links. Couns Psychol 2010;38(3):397–424.

17. Fields EL, Bogart LM, Smith KC, et al. HIV risk and perceptions of masculinity among young black men who have sex with men. J Adolesc Health 2012;50(3): 296–303.
18. Malebranche DJ, Fields EL, Bryant LO, et al. Masculine socialization and sexual risk behaviors among Black men who have sex with men: a qualitative exploration. Men Masc 2009;12(1):90–112.
19. Cross WE, Parham TA, Helms JE. The stages of Black identity development: nigrescence models. In: Jones R, editor. Black psychology. Berkeley (CA): Cobb & Henry Publishers; 1991. p. 319–38.
20. Cross WE. The psychology of nigrescence: revising the cross model. In: Ponterotto JG, Casas JM, editors. Handbook of multicultural counseling. Thousand Oaks (CA): Sage; 1995. p. 93–122.
21. Martinez DG, Sullivan SC. African American gay men and lesbians: examining the complexity of gay identity development. J Hum Behav Soc Environ 1998; 1(2/3):243–64.
22. Whitehead TL, Peterson JL, Kaljee L. The "hustle": socioeconomic deprivation, urban drug trafficking, and low-income, African-American male gender identity. Pediatrics 1994;93(6):1050–4.
23. Frable DE, Platt L, Hoey S. Concealable stigmas and positive self-perceptions: feeling better around similar others. J Pers Soc Psychol 1998;74(4):909–22.
24. Nesmith AA, Burton DL, Cosgrove TJ. Gay, lesbian, and bisexual youth and young adults: social support in their own words. J Homosex 1999;37:95–108.
25. Zimmerman L, Darnell DA, Rhew IC, et al. Resilience in community: a social ecological development model for young adult sexual minority women. Am J Community Psychol 2015;55(0):179–90.
26. Connell RW. Masculinities. Berkeley (CA): University of California Press; 1995.
27. Majors RG, Billson JM. Cool pose: the dilemmas of black manhood in America. Lexington (MA): DC Heath and Co; 1992.
28. Hunter AG, Davis JE. Hidden voices of black men: the meaning, structure, and complexity of manhood. J Black Stud 1994;25(1):20–40.
29. Stokes JP, Peterson JL. Homophobia, self-esteem, and risk for HIV among African American men who have sex with men. AIDS Educ Prev 1998;10(3):278–92.
30. Quinn K, Dickson-Gomez J. Homonegativity, religiosity, and the intersecting identities of young black men who have sex with men. AIDS Behav 2015;20(1):51–64.
31. Ward EG. Homophobia, hypermasculinity and the US black church. Cult Health Sex 2005;7(5):493–504.
32. Fields EL, Bogart LM, Smith KC, et al. "I always felt I had to prove my manhood": homosexuality, masculinity, gender role strain, and HIV risk among young black men who have sex with men. Am J Public Health 2015;105(1):122–31.
33. Balaji AB, Oster AM, Viall AH, et al. Role flexing: how community, religion, and family shape the experiences of young black men who have sex with men. AIDS Patient Care STDS 2012;26(12):730–7.
34. Hackney CH, Sanders GS. Religiosity and mental health: a meta–analysis of recent studies. J Sci Study Relig 2003;42(1):43–55.
35. Powell LH, Shahabi L, Thoresen CE. Religion and spirituality: linkages to physical health. Am Psychol 2003;58(1):36–52.
36. Barnes DM, Meyer IH. Religious affiliation, internalized homophobia, and mental health in lesbians, gay men, and bisexuals. Am J Orthop 2012;82(4):505–15.
37. Meyer IH. Minority stress and mental health in gay men. J Health Soc Behav 1995;36:38–56.

38. Herek GM, Norton AT, Allen TJ, et al. Demographic, psychological, and social characteristics of self-identified lesbian, gay, and bisexual adults in a US probability sample. Sex Res Social Policy 2010;7(3):176–200.
39. Lincoln CE, Mamiya LH. The black church in the African American experience. Durham (NC): Duke University Press; 1990.
40. Fullilove MT, Fullilove RE. Stigma as an obstacle to AIDS action: the case of the African American community. Am Behav Sci 1999;42(7):1117–29.
41. Sahgal N, Smith G. A religious portrait of African Americans. in the pew forum on religion and public life. 2009. Available at: http://pewforum.org/A-Religious-Portrait-of-African-Americans.aspx. Accessed August 14, 2016.
42. Taylor RJ, Chatters LM, Jayakody R, et al. Black and white differences in religious participation: a multisample comparison. J Sci Study Relig 1996;35(4):403–10.
43. Wilcox C, Gomez L. Religion, group identification, and politics among American Blacks. Sociol Relig 1990;51(3):271–85.
44. Griffin H. Their own received them not: African American lesbians and gays in black churches. Theolog Sex 2000;6(12):88–100.
45. Arnett JJ. Emerging adulthood: the winding road from the late teens through the twenties. Oxford University Press; 2014.
46. Pitt RN. "Still Looking for my Jonathan": Gay Black Men's management of religious and sexual identity conflicts. J Homosex 2009;57(1):39–53.
47. Winder TA. "Shouting it out": religion and the development of black gay identities. Qual Sociol 2015;38(4):375–94.
48. Mustanski B, Birkett M, Kuhns LM, et al. The role of geographic and network factors in racial disparities in HIV among young men who have sex with men: an egocentric network study. AIDS Behav 2015;19(6):1037–47.
49. Koblin BA, Mayer KH, Eshleman SH, et al. Correlates of HIV acquisition in a cohort of Black men who have sex with men in the United States: HIV prevention trials network (HPTN) 061. PLoS One 2013;8(7):e70413.
50. Lillie-Blanton M, Laveist T. Race/ethnicity, the social environment, and health. Soc Sci Med 1996;43(1):83–91.
51. Steptoe A, Feldman PJ. Neighborhood problems as sources of chronic stress: development of a measure of neighborhood problems, and associations with socioeconomic status and health. Ann Behav Med 2001;23(3):177–85.
52. Auerbach JD, Parkhurst JO, Cáceres CF. Addressing social drivers of HIV/AIDS for the long-term response: conceptual and methodological considerations. Glob Public Health 2011;6(Suppl 3):S293–309.
53. Browning CR, Burrington LA, Leventhal T, et al. Neighborhood structural inequality, collective efficacy, and sexual risk behavior among urban youth. J Health Soc Behav 2008;49(3):269–85.
54. Huebner DM, Kegeles SM, Rebchook GM, et al. Social oppression, psychological vulnerability, and unprotected intercourse among young Black men who have sex with men. Health Psychol 2014;33(12):1568.
55. Eaton LA, Driffin DD, Bauermeister J, et al. Minimal awareness and stalled uptake of pre-exposure prophylaxis (PrEP) among at risk, HIV-negative, black men who have sex with men. AIDS Patient Care STDS 2015;29(8):423–9.
56. Millett GA, Peterson JL, Wolitski RJ, et al. Greater risk for HIV infection of black men who have sex with men: a critical literature review. Am J Public Health 2006;96(6):1007–19.
57. Williams DR, Collins C. Racial residential segregation: a fundamental cause of racial disparities in health. Public Health Rep 2001;116(5):404–16.

58. Raymond HF, Chen YH, Syme SL, et al. The role of individual and neighborhood factors: HIV acquisition risk among high-risk populations in San Francisco. AIDS Behav 2014;18(2):346–56.

59. Jennings JM, Reilly ML, Perin J, et al. Sex partner meeting places over time among newly HIV-diagnosed men who have sex with men in Baltimore, Maryland. Sex Transm Dis 2015;42(10):549–53.

60. Millett GA, Flores SA, Peterson JL, et al. Explaining disparities in HIV infection among black and white men who have sex with men: a meta-analysis of HIV risk behaviors. AIDS 2007;21(15):2083–91.

61. Oster AM, Wiegand RE, Sionean C, et al. Understanding disparities in HIV infection between black and white MSM in the United States. AIDS 2011;25(8):1103–12.

62. Sullivan PS, Rosenberg ES, Sanchez TH, et al. Explaining racial disparities in HIV incidence in black and white men who have sex with men in Atlanta, GA: a prospective observational cohort study. Ann Epidemiol 2015;25(6):445–54.

63. Amirkhanian Y. Social networks, sexual networks and HIV risk in men who have sex with men. Curr HIV/AIDS Rep 2014;11(1):81–92.

64. Fields E, Fullilove R, Fullilove M. HIV sexual risk taking behavior among young black MSM: Contextual factors. In 128th American Public Health Association Annual Meeting. Boston (MA), November 12-16, 2000.

65. Jerome RC, Halkitis PN. Stigmatization, stress, and the search for belonging in black men who have sex with men who use methamphetamine. J Black Psychol 2009;35(3):343–65.

66. Kraft JM, Beeker C, Stokes JP, et al. Finding the "community" in community-level HIV/AIDS interventions: formative research with young African American men who have sex with men. Health Educ Behav 2000;27(4):430–41.

67. Raymond HF, McFarland W. Racial mixing and HIV risk among men who have sex with men. AIDS Behav 2009;13(4):630–7.

68. Arrington-Sanders R, Oidtman J, Morgan A, et al. Intersecting identities in black gay and bisexual young men: a potential framework for HIV risk. J Adolesc Health 2015;56(2):S7–8.

69. Newcomb ME, Mustanski B. Internalized homophobia and internalizing mental health problems: A meta-analytic review. Clin Psychol Rev 2010;30(8):1019–29.

70. Berg RC, Munthe-Kaas HM, Ross MW. Internalized homonegativity: a systematic mapping review of empirical research. J Homosex 2016;63(4):541–58.

71. Shoptaw S, Weiss RE, Munjas B, et al. Homonegativity, substance use, sexual risk behaviors, and HIV status in poor and ethnic men who have sex with men in Los Angeles. J Urban Health 2009;86(1):77–92.

72. Wilson PA, Valera P, Martos AJ, et al. Contributions of qualitative research in informing HIV/AIDS interventions targeting black MSM in the United States. J Sex Res 2015;53(6):1–13.

73. Crawford I, Allison KW, Zamboni BD, et al. The influence of dual-identity development on the psychosocial functioning of African-American gay and bisexual men. J Sex Res 2002;39(3):179–89.

74. Kennamer JD, Honnold J, Bradford J, et al. Differences in disclosure of sexuality among African American and White gay/bisexual men: Implications for HIV/AIDS prevention. AIDS Educ Prev 2000;12(6):519.

75. Herek GM, Gillis JR, Cogan JC. Internalized stigma among sexual minority adults: insights from a social psychological perspective. J Couns Psychol 2009;56(1):32.

76. Bennett GG, Wolin KY, Robinson EL, et al. Perceived racial/ethnic harassment and tobacco use among African American young adults. Am J Public Health 2005;95(2):238–40.

77. Hussen SA, Harper GW, Bauermeister JA, et al. Psychosocial influences on engagement in care among HIV-Positive young black gay/bisexual and other men who have sex with men. AIDS Patient Care STDS 2015;29(2):77–85.

78. Arnold EA, Rebchook GM, Kegeles SM. 'Triply cursed': racism, homophobia and HIV-related stigma are barriers to regular HIV testing, treatment adherence and disclosure among young Black gay men. Cult Health Sex 2014;16(6):710–22.

79. Meyer IH. Prejudice, social stress, and mental health in lesbian, gay, and bisexual populations: conceptual issues and research evidence. Psychol Bull 2003; 129(5):674.

80. Haile R, Rowell-Cunsolo TL, Parker EA, et al. An empirical test of racial/ethnic differences in perceived racism and affiliation with the gay community: implications for HIV risk. J Soc Issues 2014;70(2):342–59.

81. Arrington-Sanders R, Harper GW, Morgan A, et al. The role of sexually explicit material in the sexual development of same-sex-attracted Black adolescent males. Arch Sex Behav 2015;44(3):597–608.

82. Fields EL, Morgan AR, Malebranche DJ, et al. The role of virtual venues among young black men who have sex with men (YBMSM): exploration of patterns of use from 2001-2011. J Adolesc Health 2015;2(56):S118–9.

83. Cohen S. Social relationships and health. Am Psychol 2004;59(8):676–84.

84. Ayala G, Bingham T, Kim J, et al. Modeling the impact of social discrimination and financial hardship on the sexual risk of HIV among Latino and black men who have sex with men. Am J Public Health 2012;102(S2):S242–9.

85. Herek GM, Garnets LD. Sexual orientation and mental health. Annu Rev Clin Psychol 2007;3(1):353–75.

86. Dupree D, Spencer TR, Spencer MB. Stigma, stereotypes and resilience identities: the relationship between identity processes and resilience processes among black American adolescents. In: Theron CL, Liebenberg L, Ungar M, editors. Youth resilience and culture: commonalities and complexities. Dordrecht (Netherlands): Springer; 2015. p. 117–29.

87. Walker JNJ, Longmire-Avital B, Golub S. Racial and sexual identities as potential buffers to risky sexual behavior for black gay and bisexual emerging adult men. Health Psychol 2014;34(8):841–6.

88. Garofalo R, Kuhns LM, Hidalgo M, et al. Impact of religiosity on the sexual risk behaviors of young men who have sex with men. J Sex Res 2015;52(5):590–8.

89. Detrie PM, Lease SH. The relation of social support, connectedness, and collective self-esteem to the psychological well-being of lesbian, gay, and bisexual youth. J Homosex 2007;53(4):173–99.

90. Frost DM, Meyer IH. Measuring community connectedness among diverse sexual minority populations. J Sex Res 2012;49(1):36–49.

91. Arnold EA, Bailey MM. Constructing home and family: how the ballroom community supports African American GLBTQ youth in the face of HIV/AIDS. J Gay Lesbian Soc Serv 2009;21(2–3):171–88.

92. Courtenay WH. Constructions of masculinity and their influence on men's well-being: a theory of gender and health. Soc Sci Med 2000;50(10):1385–401.

93. Wickman ME, Anderson NLR, Smith Greenberg C. The adolescent perception of invincibility and its influence on teen acceptance of health promotion strategies. J Pediatr Nurs 2008;23(6):460–8.

94. Institute of Medicine (IOM). Unequal treatment: confronting racial and ethnic disparities in health care. In: Smedley BD, Stith AY, Nelson AR, editors. Washington, DC: The National Academies Press; 2003. p. 782.

95. Institute of Medicine (IOM). The health of lesbian, gay, bisexual, and transgender people: building a foundation for better understanding. Washington, DC: The National Academies Press; 2011. p. 368.

96. Weissman JS, Stern R, Fielding SL, et al. Delayed access to health care: risk factors, reasons, and consequences. Ann Intern Med 1991;114(4):325–31.

97. Malmgren JA, Martin ML, Nicola RM. Health care access of poverty-level older adults in subsidized public housing. Public Health Rep 1996;111(3):260–3.

98. Malebranche DJ, Peterson JL, Fullilove RE, et al. Race and sexual identity: perceptions about medical culture and healthcare among Black men who have sex with men. J Natl Med Assoc 2004;96(1):97.

Lesbian, Gay, Bisexual, and Transgender Families

Cecil R. Webster Jr, MD*, Cynthia J. Telingator, MD

KEYWORDS

- LGBT parents • Children with LGBT parents • Microaggressions
- Assisted reproduction • LGBT parents and the health care system
- Race and ethnicity in LGBT families • Transgender parents and well-being
- Child and adolescent development in LGBT families

KEY POINTS

- Sexual minority families face unique barriers to care and health equity in health care and educational systems, as well as health-related law and policy.
- Health care providers can play an important role in navigating the unique barriers and challenges that sexual minority families face when seeking welcoming and affirming clinical practices.
- Empirical data demonstrate good functioning in the majority of children of same-sex parents.
- These children develop and function comparably to those from traditional families, and develop particular strengths that are linked to having parents who are sexual minorities.
- Familiarity with lesbian, gay, bisexual, and transgender language, family composition, support, financial vulnerability, and intersectionality with factors such as race/ethnicity are key to competency in assisting these families in the health care system.

There is a significant number of youth in families headed by sexual minorities.[1–3] Between 1.1 and 2 million children under 18 years of age have a single lesbian, gay, or bisexual parent.[2] Further, about 210,000 children are being raised by a same-sex couple, one-third (34%) of whom were married as of 2013.[3] In states that allowed same-sex marriage in 2013, just more than one-half (51%) of children raised by same-sex couples had married parents. The Institute of Medicine has identified provider knowledge about sexual minority patients, and the impact of stigma on sexual minorities' health, as areas requiring further attention.[1] Both external stigma and internalized shame may represent significant barriers to care and health equity for these families. Given the vulnerabilities of these families, and the likelihood that they are

Disclosure Statement: The authors have nothing to disclose.
Division of Child and Adolescent Psychiatry, Cambridge Health Alliance, Harvard Medical School, 1493 Cambridge Street, Cambridge, MA, USA
* Corresponding author. 137 Newbury Street, 6th Floor, Boston, MA 02116.
E-mail address: mail@cecilwebstermd.com

Pediatr Clin N Am 63 (2016) 1107–1119
http://dx.doi.org/10.1016/j.pcl.2016.07.010
0031-3955/16/© 2016 Elsevier Inc. All rights reserved.

seeking care in pediatric practices in diverse geographic and sociocultural settings, it is the goal of this article to help the clinician consider issues relevant to these families.

Internalized homophobia is something sexual minorities may experience in a society where heterosexuality is the assumed default. Some sexual and gender minority parents may worry that their sexual minority status will have a negative impact on the children owing to the children needing to contend with having a "different" family than other children in their community.[4] However, empirical data from studies with appropriate control groups indicate resilience in youth despite such concerns. Children of same-sex couples, for example, have been found to have no differences than other children on self-reported assessments of psychological well-being (eg, self-esteem, anxiety), school outcomes (eg, grade point average, trouble in school), and measures of family relationships (eg, parental warmth, care from adults and peers).[5] There are no differences in peer relationships, self-reported substance abuse, delinquency, or peer victimization.[6,7] More important than their parents' gender is the quality of relationships that exist within families that impact teenager adjustment.[8]

FAMILY STRUCTURE

The US Supreme Court's *Obergefell v. Hodges* ruling in June 2015 that established the federal recognition of same-sex marriage may increase the estimated numbers of children raised in lesbian, gay, bisexual, transgender, and queer families. This may be owing to increased visibility of these families and uniformity in marital law, which may pave the way for more lesbian, gay, bisexual, transgender, and queer families to be married and therefore included in estimates. As it stands now, nearly 1 in 5 (19%) of same-sex couples, and single lesbians, gays, and bisexuals were raising children under the age of 18.[3,9] A greater proportion (35%) of lesbian, gay, bisexual, and transgender (LGBT)-identified individuals are raising children than might be anticipated among men and women age years 50 or younger who are living alone or with a partner or spouse.[9] Currently, the vast majority of same-sex parents are female (77%).[3] This may change as there is increased acceptance of LGBT families and of men parenting. There are some complementary data that show that 27% of female couples have children and 48% of individual lesbians have children. Gay male individuals (20%) are currently more likely to raise children than male couples (11%). Adoption and foster care are prevalent in same-sex couples in general. Same-sex couples are 4 times more likely to be raising adopted children (13% vs 3% of different-sex couples) and 6 times more likely to be raising foster children (2% vs 0.3% of different-sex couples).[9]

Family structures may change and evolve over time. Detailed demographic and related research are necessary to characterize these families, and studies may fail to capture their full diversity (eg, socioeconomic level, race, sexual orientation, and gender expression) given limits in scope, reach, and view.[1,4,10] Therefore, the information presented here may have methodologic limitations, but may nevertheless aid in understanding sexual minority parent families.

PARENTING PREPARATION

Let us consider the following vignette to guide our exploration:

Javier and Jonathan have come to your office together and are interviewing new pediatricians because they are anxiously awaiting the birth of a daughter next month. They have one 10-year-old son, Joey, from Javier's previous relationship. The two initially considered seeing Joey's pediatrician; however, they felt less confident that this physician was able to care for their family.

Assessment of their worries not only about parenthood, but also about other issues that they may be concerned about regarding work and community, can be explored. Becoming a parent in general is enough to create some anxiety, although you tactfully ask what is causing their anxiety.

Jonathan confirms that he is "the nervous one," attesting to his already perceptible worry. He states that this will be his first time caring for an infant. Javier interjects that Joey, their 10-year-old son, is his and his ex-wife's biological child. Joey joined their family 2 years ago, after a lengthy and contentious custody battle. Their previsit form lists Jonathan and Javier as married and Javier having sole legal and physical custody of Joey.

You inquire about the supports that Javier and Jonathan share and their experience of these changes in their family.

Jonathan says that he worries about Javier's parents and brother, members of his religiously conservative family in Guatemala. They have not been accepting of their marriage, and have coolly received their decision to have a child through surrogacy. In contrast, Javier's sister has been helpful in navigating stroller choices and preschools. Jonathan's family organized their gender-atypical Tonka Truck–themed baby shower last month. Jonathan tears up as he intimates that he never thought he would have the chance to be "a real dad," but worries about the stares he gets in the grocery store as an African American caring for a light-complexioned Latin child. Javier clasps his hand and offers a light quip about their "Modern Family." Although their 10-year-old, Joey, has adjusted decently, both men ask you if their daughter and Joey will be alright?

One may infer that Javier and Jonathan may experience exclusion. Concerns about the impact on their children not being raised in a heterosexual family not only exists within their extended family, stigmas they may experience owing to rejection from their community and religious organizations may also impact them. The impact of growing up with sexual minority parents should neither be underemphasized nor overemphasized.[8] Children of sexual minority parents develop in ways that are typical and healthy.[11,12] Many parents may grapple with their own experiences of shame and stigma that they have endured "coming out." They may face more experiences of stigmatization as they move toward parenthood. Worries of prospective LGBT parents may include concerns about whether or not their children will experience rejection based on the parent's/parents' sexual orientation.[13] Although many sexual minorities were raised in welcoming environments, many others have experienced consistent rejection for being different from others; this feeling may continue to resonate in their transition to parenthood. Further, they may experience a paucity of sources of social support in the process of becoming parents.

A second no less important factor with stigma involves race and ethnicity (see Errol Fields and colleagues' article, "The intersection of sociocultural factors and health-related behavior in LGBT youth: Experiences among young black gay males as an example," in this issue). This is a layer that is often overlooked in clinical discussions related to sexuality and gender identity. Kimberlyn Leary, PhD, has offered the clinical concept of 'racial enactments,' or sequences of our cultural attitudes and actions toward race and racial differences. She postulates that America's most significant racial enactment has been a relative silence about racial issues.[14] Creating a relationship in which the role of race and ethnicity is included in the dialogue of assessing the needs of LGBT families' is important. For example, it may be wise to ask families about how their race/ethnicity or national origin may affect their relationship with schools, family, and community.

Identity is complex. The status of being sexual and ethnic minorities may compete.[15] There may be stigmatization of ethnic minorities within the LGBT community, and conversely homophobic stigmatization within their ethnic community. It has been found that African Americans, for example, are less involved in gay and lesbian communities. Similarly, African Americans and Latinos tend to disclose their sexual orientation less often.[15] Therefore, these populations may not readily reveal their gender or sexual differences in school and work environments. These dual identities of being both an ethnic as well as a sexual minority may create barriers to pediatric care, cause isolation from sources of family and community support and constitute a special population that is not always specifically addressed in the research literature.

Sexual minority families exist in all regions of the United States.[3] Overall numbers of same-sex couples (both those with and without children) does not vary greatly by region (18% of same-sex couples live in the Northeast, Midwest, and South; 17% in the West). However, the subset of same-sex couples with children are more likely to live in certain regions as compared with different-sex couples with children. They are more likely to live in the Northeast (34% vs 17%) and West (29% vs 24%) in comparison to traditional couples with children.[3] It is unclear if this is related to greater protections of antidiscrimination laws, greater availability of marriage equality laws in the Northeast and West as of 2013, or cultural differences across regions.

Laws related to adoption, health care, and workplace discrimination as they pertain to sexual minorities are changing. Will Jonathan be able to formally adopt Joey? Is Jonathan at risk of losing his job given his sexuality? Will both parents be able to be listed on their daughter's birth certificate? The answers to these questions vary by state and statute, and are in flux at present.

For a more comprehensive view of sexual minorities raising children, it is also important to consider that lesbian, gay, and bisexuals are also raising children as members of different-sex couples. In an article published by the Williams Institute, researchers specify that of people who identified as bisexuals who are raising children, more than one-half (51%) were married to a different-sex spouse, and 11% had a different-sex unmarried partner. In contrast, only 4% had a same-sex spouse or partner. For lesbians and gay men both, 18% had a different-sex married spouse and 4% had a different-sex unmarried partner.[2] Therefore, in the waiting room or examination room, these families may not be easily identified.

Often sexual minorities conceal their identity or avoid interactions to cope with bias, and are thus vulnerable to overt or covert stigma, and ostracism. To deliver equitable health care, it is important that providers mitigate potential unnecessary barriers to care. To do so, the clinical environment and administrative interactions are as meaningful as are the clinical face-to-face experiences. For example, the use of gender-neutral terms (eg, 'parent' vs 'mother' or 'father') on forms, documents, and set-up calls for appointments can help to create a nonjudgmental and therefore welcoming health care environment[16] (see Scott E. Hadland and colleagues' article, "Caring for LGBT Youth & Families in Inclusive and Affirmative Environments," in this issue). Familiarly with the terminology related to sexual orientation and gender, and comfort addressing the various pathways to LGBT parenthood, can promote openness and a positive clinical alliance with diverse families within a pediatric practice (**Box 1**).

Asking what is an individual's preferred name and pronoun may prove helpful in reducing barriers to health care. These barriers may affect those who are not recognized to be transgender or have gender variant identities. A small Canadian study

---

Box 1
Office preparation

Verbal

- Use of gender neutral terms (eg, 'parent' vs 'mother,' 'father').
- Inquiring how the parent would like to be addressed (eg, 'co-mother,' 'dad').
- Ease of use of sexual orientation and gender language with staff and clinicians.
- Familiarity and use of pathways to parenthood language.

Nonverbal

- Forms with gender neutral terms (eg, 'parent 1,' 'parent 2').
- Rainbow flags, pins, magnets or other LGBT-friendly symbols visible.
- Nondiscrimination policies featured prominently.
- Inclusive language on printed materials, forms, and online presence.
- Frequent checking in with yourself and staff about heterosexual assumptions.

---

about the interaction that transgender adults and their partners had with assisted reproduction clinics noted that staff and clinicians incorrectly assumed that they were cisgender heterosexual couples, and encouraged them to conceive naturally. The data surrounding the experience of transgender parents in health care settings is modest, but 1 study found that the use of gender neutral terms such as 'parent,' warmth of and supportive interactions with providers, and familiarly with transgender terms may be helpful.[17] The study noted problems with clinical documentation, requiring patients to alter gender terms on their forms, as well as refusals of services.[17] Creating a welcoming environment helps to foster clinical alliances with all families.

Visible cues and signs of nondiscriminatory practices both online and in the office may be help to convey a safe environment for sexual minority families. Depending on the setting, these might include symbols of LGBT equality (appropriate waiting room information or literature, "safe space" or "rainbow" symbols, etc). Staff and clinician ease with questions that pertain to sexual minority families may also help to communicate a clear willingness to provide professional care to all, and an openness to hear their unique needs. All families respond to the environment in which they seek care. Creating a nonstigmatizing professional space is 1 way to make families feel more comfortable. Setting an environment where the family may discuss and disclose their family constellation freely is ideal.[8]

PATHWAYS TO PARENTHOOD

Sexual minorities are 3 times more likely to be raising adopted children as compared with heterosexual couples, and the number of same-sex couples pursuing adoption has doubled in the last 10 years.[3,4] In addition, sexual minority parents are more likely to complete interracial adoptions,[18] half of children of same-sex couples are nonwhite,[2] and a significant portion of same-sex couples with children are nonwhite.[2,3]

Although a large portion of same-sex couples are raising adopted or foster children, most (51%) of the children in a same-sex couple are identified as the biological child of 1 parent.[3] There are few data outlining what proportion of these children include parents from a previous heterosexual relationship.

Javier and Jonathan explain that it was a difficult decision, but chose to use Jonathan's sperm because he had not fathered a biologically related child in contrast with Javier. The two explain that it may be easier at kindergarten pickup to have a child that may plausibly be related to either of them, so they elected to use egg donation as part of their expanding family. They have not decided if they will tell the whole family immediately.

Assisted reproductive technology, a medical intervention used by many heterosexual as well as LGBT families and which Javier and Jonathan have elected, broadly includes all fertility treatments in which both sperm and eggs are handled. In general, this may include removing eggs from ovaries, combining them with sperm in a laboratory, and implanting them in a uterus. In regards to eggs and sperm, there are 3 main types of donors in assisted reproductive technology (**Box 2**), although this list is not exhaustive. In the known identity donor type (eg, an in-law, sibling, friend), a donor may serve as a parent, "aunt," family friend, or another arrangement.[8] Second, there is the open identity donor. In this arrangement, the donor agrees to allow contact at a certain age (often when the child reaches 18).[19] The third is an unknown donor. In these cases, the donor remains forever anonymous to the recipient and child.[8]

Gay men may elect to have biologically related children. One man may use sperm to attempt to conceive or the 2 men may combine their sperm to attempt to conceive. Surrogacy may involve 1 woman (for both egg donation and surrogacy) or 2 women (1 for egg donation, and another for surrogacy). Agencies may assist gay couples with choosing egg donors, surrogates, and fertility clinics.[8] One study of 15 gay male couples recruited in a fertility center in Connecticut went deeper in outlining what the participants regarded as important considerations for male same-sex couples looking toward surrogacy.[20] These considerations included relationship stability, medical/legal demands, family support, sperm decisions, egg donor and gestational carrier choices, and disclosure to children.[20]

Lesbian couples often elect insemination, or less often donor eggs from known, open-identity, or unknown donors according to preferences and circumstance.[8,19] One member of the couple may serve as biological parent or birthing parent. One may carry the child conceived with their partner's egg. In a couple each woman may elect to conceive so that both have the opportunity give birth.[8] These are examples of options and should not be considered comprehensive.

One study of 129 lesbian mothers and 77 offspring recruited nationwide through the US National Longitudinal Lesbian Family Study sought to get a greater understanding of parent satisfaction in donor choice 18 years after conception. The authors of this study acknowledge that a limitation of this study was that the respondents were mostly white, urban, and middle class; however, it broadens our knowledge of sexual minority families in general that have used assisted reproduction.[19]

Of the mothers in this study, 36.4% chose known donors, 24.7% open identity donors, and 39% unknown donors. Those that were satisfied with their choice of donor

---

Box 2
Assisted reproduction donor types

Known identity donor: Egg or sperm donor is known to the family; often friend, in-law, or sibling.

Open identity donor: Egg or sperm donor agrees to allow contact at a certain age (often when the child reaches 18).

Unknown donor: Egg or sperm donor remains forever anonymous to the family.

type were spread nearly equally between all groups; however, of those that were dissatisfied with their choice, the majority had used unknown donors. Often, they noted that this dissatisfaction surrounded the mothers' desire that their children have information or access to the donor. Interestingly, satisfaction was not related to their child's psychological health, as assessed by the anxiety, anger, and depression subscales of the State-Trait Personality Inventory. Previous studies have outlined that donor type (ie, known identity, open identity, or unknown identity) had no influence on quality of life or psychological adjustment for adolescents. The mother's feelings about donor access, and custody concerns played central roles in this satisfaction or lack thereof.[19]

Despite the increased prevalence of media representations of transgender individuals and parents, and the Institute of Medicine's identification of transgender-specific health research as a need, information regarding this population of parents is scant.[1,21] As a part of the survey phase of a Canadian Institutes of Health Research-funded community-based study of the health and well-being, 1 study from Ontario, Canada, surveyed 110 transgender parents. The authors found that nearly one-quarter (24.1%) of transgender adults in Ontario are parents and a significant majority of them (77.9%) reported that they were biological parents to their children. The desire to have more children was reported in 19.4% of the transgender parents and 36.7% of the transgender nonparents.[21]

Transgender adults who will undergo gender-affirming treatments, including hormone therapy or sex reassignment surgery, may choose to ensure future parenthood in several ways. Transgender women (ie, born male sex, now identifying as female) may elect to have cryopreservation of sperm. Transgender men (ie, born female sex, now identifying as a man) may elect cryopreservation of ovarian tissue. This may be performed during the removal of 1 or both ovaries, thus alleviating the need for invasive follicle stimulation later.[21]

One can imagine that inquiring about how Javier and Jonathan chose to be parents, which, if either, parent offered donor material and why, and their satisfaction, and perception of their child's well-being thus far may be critical elements in appraising their family's needs.

Overall, sexual minority adults may have many paths to parenthood. There is a great diversity of ethnic, social, economic, religious, and family culture with the community of families headed by sexual minorities. Much current research has heavily used white, urban, and female populations. Our general understanding of these families and their needs may become more roundly elucidated with additional research attention to the robust populations of families that exist outside of those characteristics (see Errol Fields and colleagues' article, "The intersection of sociocultural factors and health-related behavior in LGBT youth: Experiences among young black gay males as an example," in this issue).

CHILDHOOD AND PARENTHOOD

Considerations for follow-up appointments after an initial meeting often include routine questions about parenting. In discussions with individual family members, especially privacy conscious youth, reviewing confidentiality is important to establish a sense of safety to discuss all family members' concerns and needs.[22] Clinicians should remember that, because of stigma, that members of families headed by sexual minority parents can experience, an assessment of bullying experienced by youth in these families should be a included in discussions with and about them.[15,23]

At their follow-up visit, Javier and Jonathan ask not about their arriving daughter, but about their 10-year-old son, Joey, who accompanies them.

Javier feels that he and his ex-wife have managed well with Joey. Javier suspects that Joey's parochial school, one Joey has attended since kindergarten and one initially chosen by Javier's then wife, has been less accommodating to the changes in the family composition to include Jonathan. Jonathan is quick to point out the frequent phone calls placed to his always available real estate office from the elementary school nurse owing to Joey's somatic complaints. Joey frequently requests to come home early from school. The 3—Javier, Jonathan, and Joey—notice that he has received a number of detentions owing to verbal altercations with others and all agree that is unusual for Joey. They mention that they have noticed Joey has participated in fewer afterschool sports in the last 2 years. He seldom has friends over after school in contrast with his previously busy social calendar, despite living 2 blocks from the school. The fathers suspect that other parents and school administration are either unsure how to interact with their family regarding an increasing number of athletic and other peer activities, or reluctant to do so. They indicate that they have tried to prepare Joey that others may not understand their family composition. They wonder if the stigma of having gay parents is impacting Joey.

Stigma can be a contributing factor in health and mental health morbidity; therefore, it can be helpful for the pediatrician to assess parent perceptions of community and school support. It is no less important to explore the child's perspective, which may be complementary and/or contrasting (**Box 3**). Subtle and not-so-subtle social ostracism may manifest stigmatization, and may adversely impact children in a variety of ways (see Valerie A. Earnshaw and colleagues' article, "LGBT Youth and Bullying," in this issue).

One study showed that, of children with LGBT parents, 23% reported feeling unsafe at school because of their unique family constellation, 40% reported being harassed in school because of their family, and 23% reported mistreatment and negative remarks by their peers' parents.[24] It is important that families be encouraged to discuss any concerns they may have about such experiences, and that their children be included equally in school and community protections against bullying or harassment. Otherwise, the child's sense that his or her experiences are acceptable for discussion may be adversely impacted by his or her parents' own anxiety about difficult experiences the child may be facing as a result of the parent's sexual orientation. They may also experience stigmatization in school settings and develop consequent shame. In such circumstances, instead of discussing any concerns appropriately, children may misperceive that there is something negative or wrong with them, and internalize this stigma,[13] a significant risk factor for poor mental health outcomes that is associated with significant morbidity and mortality.

In addition, sexual minority families and children may experience microaggressions. Microaggressions are subtle, albeit sometimes commonplace, verbal, behavioral, or environmental indignities originally studied in relation to bias and stigma regarding racial and ethnic differences.[23] In a small study of a nationwide sample of 49 children with same-sex parents, more than one-half of children reported microaggressions related to their families being same-sex parented. Most of these involved heterosexism, or behaviors or interactions that assume heterosexuality (eg, 'Where's your mom?' to a child with 2 fathers). Other themes included their family being publicly exposed to others' negative judgments without their consent, having to be a spokesperson for families like theirs, or having the legitimacy of their family questioned.[23]

Stigma may insidiously delegitimize LGBT families. One of 3 recent United States Supreme Court rulings affirming federal equality regarding same-sex marriage discussed this issue in relating research evidence on the well-being of youth in these

Box 3
Examination room inquiries for families

Opening questions

- Who is in your family?
- How would you prefer to be addressed?
- Tell me about your family?
- Are there other individuals that assist in parenting?
- Who are the major caretakers in your child's life?

Parenthood inquiries

- Tell me about your relationship with one another.
- How did you decide to become parents?
- What is your child's awareness of your path to parenthood? Your family's? Your community's? Do you anticipate this will change in the future?
- What do your children call you at home?
- How did you decide on who would have a genetic link to your child?
- Could you tell me about the birth and pregnancy with your child?
- How has your adjustment to parenthood been?
- What are the current roles of the donors?
- Who share legal or custodial responsibilities for your child?
- Are there any legal or custody concerns?
- Tell me about the role of race/ethnicity in your child's life. Have there been challenges?
- What or who are the supports in your family? Do you feel supported?
- Are you a member of a religious community? What is that relationship like?
- Is your family financially vulnerable?
- What would you like to get most out of our time together today?

Child inquiries

- How did your family form?
- Your parents explained a lot. What is the rest of the story?
- Sometimes families feel different. Does yours?
- What do you love about your family?
- Do others treat your family differently? How so?
- Do you feel safe in school?
- Who are the important adults in your life? Who do you go to when you have a problem? When you have something you're proud of?
- Are there things about your family that you worry about?
- What are the other important things I should know about you?

families to society's interest in preventing the known potential harm of stigma to both them and their parents:

> *A third basis for protecting the right to marry is that it safeguards children and families and thus draws meaning from related rights of childrearing, procreation, and education....Without the recognition, stability, and predictability marriage offers, children suffer the stigma of knowing their families are somehow lesser. They also suffer the significant material costs of being raised by unmarried parents, relegated to a more difficult and uncertain family life. The marriage laws at issue thus harm and humiliate the children of same-sex couples.*[25]

Relating this to the previous vignette, although it is unclear whether or not job instability or economic vulnerability is present for Joey's family, it is an important issue to assess in families headed by sexual minorities. Because poverty and single parenthood are important risk factors for a variety of adverse health and developmental outcomes, pediatric health care providers should be aware that many LGBT families face these disadvantages and are economically vulnerable.[2,3] Single LGBT adults raising children are 3 times as likely as comparable non-LGBT individuals to have household incomes near the poverty threshold.[2] Being coupled or married is associated with a decreased but still significant risk for poverty. Married or unmarried LGBT individuals in a 2-adult household with children are twice as likely as comparable non-LGBT individuals to have household incomes near the poverty threshold.[2]

Interestingly, there are some economic differences noted between families with married and unmarried same-sex couples. The Williams Institute analyzed demographic data of the US Census Bureau's 2013 American Community Survey, the first national demographic survey to explicitly include married and unmarried same-sex couples. Their analysis revealed that when raised by married same-sex couples, an average of only 9% of children are in households near the poverty line versus 11% of their peers in different-sex families.[3] In general, however, the median annual household income of both married and unmarried same-sex couples with children is lower than that of different-sex couples ($75,000 vs $79,200 respectively).[3] In short, having married same-sex parents puts children at decreased but still significant risk of poverty than the children of married different-sex parents, and the incomes of same-sex couples are lower.[3]

Further, children of same-sex parents are less likely to have private health insurance than their peers with married opposite-sex parents.[26] This difference is diminished in states with legal same-sex marriage and civil unions or second-parent adoptions for gay and lesbian couples. Because federal marriage equality laws lead to greater uniformity in adoption and health laws locally, these differences between LGBT families and the general population may diminish. What is clear is that, outside of marriage, there is significant economic vulnerability in these families and less access to private health insurance.

More information is needed about the household incomes of couples that elect costly fertility assistance versus adoptions or those who have biological children from previous relationships. Also information is needed about the income of ethnic minorities that are parents and the potentially related economic disadvantages. For the family of Joey, a loss of a job may mean the loss of private insurance and the access to care it provides.

Apart from these economic issues, helping children to cope with the harmful effects of anti-LGBT family stigma reflecting the opinion that "their families are somehow lesser" mentioned in the Supreme Court decision is a typical concern unique to the experience of LGBT families. Fortunately for children, coping factors such as having positive concepts of their families seems to confer resilience that mitigates the risks of stigma associated with the marginalization that some children experience.[23] In a small study of a nationwide sample of 49 children with same-sex parents, positive conceptualizations of these children's families were expressed more frequently and rated at a medium or high salience by nearly three-quarters (71%) of the respondents. In contrast, those expressing experiencing microaggressions (57%) or feelings of difference (78%) were typically at a low or medium salience with neutral (rather than negative) emotion. In other words, these experiences of microaggressions and feelings of difference may not have been particularly significant to them, suggesting that their positive conceptions may confer resilience to anti-LGBT minority stress.[23]

For these reasons, overt and covert stigma may burden many children being raised in LGBT families. Race and economics are important additional factors to consider in a clinical interaction, as they are powerful risk factors for adverse health and developmental outcomes (see Errol Fields and colleagues' article, "The intersection of sociocultural factors and health-related behavior in LGBT youth: Experiences among young black gay males as an example," in this issue).

SUMMARY

Recent research paints an increasingly rich portrait of sexual minority-parented families. However, despite recent changes in laws, policies, and social attitudes leading to greater visibility, acceptance, and equality of LGBT families, they still face some unique difficulties in the health care, school, and legal systems. At the population level, group-level point estimates in studies to date indicate that children raised by same-sex couples develop and function comparably to the general population. At the individual or family level, however, risk factors such as stigma may confer risk. Health care providers are in a position to assist families navigate unique barriers with some welcoming and relevant clinical practices.

Much research to date has used nonpopulation samples that are relatively small, white, affluent, and urban, which is not representative of the true ethnic, socioeconomic, and geographic diversity of sexual minority families. Robust research has been conducted on children raised by lesbian mothers; more research is needed on children raised by gay fathers and transgender parents. Data on transgender parents and children of transgender parents are particularly sparse and an important research need, as is gathering more data on LGBT parents and their children in diverse communities. Reliable and valid population-based studies capturing the diversity of LGBT families is needed.

These families are multidimensional and not reducible to a collection of data. Familiarity with language concerning sexual minorities, and an attentive ear to family composition and experience is an important foundation for a competent clinical alliance. Clear assessments of networks of support and financial vulnerability may be helpful in understanding the family's needs. Awareness of community and online programs and supports for families can also be extremely helpful. In addition, sensitive exploration of the important dimension of race and ethnicity in double minority populations is important.

Many sexual minority families may not identify themselves as such, and may not be recognized clinically. Bisexual parents in different-sex couples, single gay and lesbian parents, and transgender parents in seemingly opposite-sex relationships may not be readily identifiable. It is important to cultivate a welcoming and safe office and clinical environment that facilitates disclosure of the patient's family constellation.

Much of the research described above preceded the June 2015 *Obergefell v Hodges* Supreme Court decision guaranteeing same-sex couples the right to marry nationwide. Future studies may have the opportunity to review potential changes in marriage rates, family composition economic stability, and use of health insurance, all of which may conceivably be impacted by same-sex marriage availability. In addition, shifting cultural attitudes regarding same-sex marriage may facilitate needed research on same-sex parenthood.

As sexual minority families become more visible and diversified, their health needs may shift. As health care providers, pediatricians and allied professionals have opportunities to anticipate and navigate these shifting challenges for LGBT families, and provide them the safe and competent care.

REFERENCES

1. Institute of Medicine. The health of lesbian, gay, bisexual, and transgender people: building a foundation for better understanding. Washington, DC: The National Academies Press; 2011.
2. Gates GJ. LGB families and relationships: analyses of the 2013 National Health Interview Survey. Los Angeles (CA): The Williams Institute; 2014. Available at: http://williamsinstitute.law.ucla.edu/research/census-lgbt-demographics-studies/lgb-families-nhis-sep-2014/. Accessed November 9, 2015.
3. Gates GJ. Demographics of married and unmarried same sex couples: analyses of the 2013 American Community Survey. Los Angeles (CA): The Williams Institute; 2015. Available at: http://williamsinstitute.law.ucla.edu/research/census-lgbt-demographics-studies/demographics-of-married-and-unmarried-same-sex-couples-analyses-of-the-2013-american-community-survey/. Accessed November 9, 2015.
4. Goldberg A. Lesbian and gay parents and their children: research on the family life cycle. In: Introduction: lesbian and gay parents and their children-research and contemporary issues. Washington, DC: American Psychological Association; 2010. p. 3–14.
5. Wainright J, Russell S, Patterson C. Psychosocial adjustment, school outcomes, and romantic relationships of adolescents with same-sex parents. Child Dev 2004;75:1886–98.
6. Wainright J, Patterson C. Delinquency, victimization, and substance use among adolescents with female same-sex parents. J Fam Psychol 2006;20:526–30.
7. Wainright J, Patterson C. Peer relations among adolescents with female same-sex parents. Dev Psychol 2008;44:117–26.
8. Telingator C, Patterson C. Children and adolescents of lesbian and gay parents. J Am Acad Child Adolesc Psychiatry 2008;47:1364–8.
9. Gates GJ. LGBT parenting in the United States. The Williams Institute; 2013. Available at: http://williamsinstitute.law.ucla.edu/research/census-lgbt-demographics-studies/lgbt-parenting-in-the-united-states/. Accessed November 9, 2015.
10. Goldberg A, Gartrell N. LGB-parent families: the current state of the research and directions for the future. Adv Child Dev Behav 2014;46:55–88.
11. Golombok S, Mellish L, Jennings S, et al. Adoptive gay father families: parent-child relationships and children's psychological adjustment. Child Dev 2013;85:456–68.
12. van Gelderen L, Gartrell N, Bos H, et al. Stigmatization and resilience in adolescent children of lesbian mothers. J GLBT Fam Stud 2009;5:268–79.
13. Telingator C. Clinical work with children and adolescents growing up with lesbian, gay, and bisexual parents. In: Goldberg A, Allen K, editors. LGBT-Parent

families: innovations in research and implications for practice. New York: Springer New York; 2013. p. 261–74.

14. Leary K. Racial enactments in dynamic treatment. Psychoanal Dialogues 2000; 10:639–53.

15. Jamil OB, Harper GW, Fernandez M. Sexual and ethnic identity development among gay/bisexual/questioning (GBQ) male ethnic minority adolescents. Cultur Divers Ethnic Minor Psychol 2009;15:203–14.

16. Coren J. Assessing your office for care of lesbian, gay, bisexual, and transgender patients. Health Care Manag (Frederick) 2011;30:66–70.

17. James-Abraham S, Tarasoff L, Green D, et al. Trans people's experience with assisted reproductive services: a qualitative study. Hum Reprod 2015;30:1365–74.

18. Farr H, Patterson C. Transracial adoption by lesbian, gay, and heterosexual couples: who complete transracial adoptions and with what results? Adopt Q 2009; 12:187–204.

19. Gartrell N, Bos H, Goldberg N, et al. Satisfaction with known, open-identity, or unknown sperm donors: reports from lesbian mothers of 17-year-old adolescents. Fertil Steril 2015;103:242–8.

20. Greenfeld D, Seli E. Gay men choosing parenthood through assisted reproduction: medical and psychosocial considerations. Fertil Steril 2011;95:225–9.

21. Pyne J, Bauer G, Bradley K, et al. Transphobia and other stressors impacting trans parents. J GLBT Fam Stud 2015;11:107–26.

22. Adelson S, American Academy of Child and Adolescent Psychiatry Committee on Quality Issues. Practice parameter on gay, lesbian, or bisexual sexual orientation, gender nonconformity, and gender discordance in children and adolescents. J Am Acad Child Adolesc Psychiatry 2012;51:957–74.

23. Farr R, Crain E, Oakley M, et al. Microaggressions, feelings of difference, and resilience among adopted children with sexual minority parents. J Youth Adolesc 2016;45:85–104.

24. Kosciw J, Diaz E. Involved, invisible, ignored: the experiences of lesbian, gay, bisexual and transgender parents and their children in our nation's K-12 school. Gay, Lesbian and Straight Education Network; 2008. Available at: http://www.glsen.org/download/file/MzIyNg==. Accessed November 9, 2015.

25. Obergefell v. Hodges, 576 U.S.___. 2015.

26. Gonzales G, Blewett L. Disparities in health insurance among children with same-sex parents. J Pediatr 2013;132:703–11.

What the Primary Care Pediatrician Needs to Know About Gender Incongruence and Gender Dysphoria in Children and Adolescents

CrossMark

Annelou L.C. de Vries, MD, PhD[a],*, Daniel Klink, MD, PhD[b], Peggy T. Cohen-Kettenis, PhD[c]

KEYWORDS

- Gender dysphoria • Gender incongruence • Gender variance • Children
- Adolescents • Transgender care

KEY POINTS

- Many children diagnosed with gender incongruence do not become transgender adolescents or adults.
- Delaying puberty as part of multidisciplinary care can help transgender adolescents develop into well-functioning young adults.
- During medical endocrine treatment few adverse events occur, but long-term outcomes are currently unknown.
- Research evidence is limited concerning what is best transgender care for children and adolescents who have gender dysphoria; existing guidelines are consensus based.

INTRODUCTION AND TERMINOLOGY

For an ever more visible group of children and adolescents their sense of being male or female, named gender identity, is incongruent with their birth-assigned sex and sexual body characteristics. They may suffer from gender dysphoria, the distress resulting from this incongruence. These youth form a subgroup of the children and adolescents with gender variance or gender nonconformity, which refers to the entire spectrum of

The authors have nothing to disclose.
[a] Department of Child and Adolescent Psychiatry, VU University Medical Center, Room 1y130, PO Box 7057, 1007 MB Amsterdam, The Netherlands; [b] Division of Endocrinology, Department of Pediatrics, VU University Medical Center, PO Box 7057, 1007 MB Amsterdam, The Netherlands; [c] Department of Medical Psychology, VU University Medical Center, PO Box 7057, 1007 MB Amsterdam, The Netherlands
* Corresponding author.
E-mail address: alc.devries@vumc.nl

Pediatr Clin N Am 63 (2016) 1121–1135
http://dx.doi.org/10.1016/j.pcl.2016.07.011
0031-3955/16/© 2016 Elsevier Inc. All rights reserved.

variation in gender role behavior or gender expression, with or without gender identity variance, behavior that is considered nonstereotypical for one's birth-assigned sex. This group also includes many gay, lesbian, and bisexual youth without gender identity variance (See Stewart Adelson and colleagues article, "Development and Mental Health of LGBT Youth in Pediatric Practice," in this issue, for fuller discussion of multiple LGBT developmental trajectories; and the American Academy of Child and Adolescent Psychiatry Practice Parameter[1]).

Gender is not a dichotomous concept but consists of more than the male-female binary. Such terms as nonbinary, gender queer, third gender, or a-gender reflect this. Social transitioning is used when someone starts to live in the experienced gender role and encompasses clothing, gender role behavior, and the use of a name and pronouns of that gender. Gender-affirming treatment is the clinical approach that supports the expression of one's experienced gender of which puberty blockers, hormone treatment, and surgeries may be part. However, such treatments may not be desired or needed by all gender identity variant youth, some of whom do not experience distress. A transwoman is a birth-assigned male with a female gender identity, and a transman is a birth-assigned female who identifies as male. Male-to-female transgender and female-to-male transgender are also used terms.

Gender dysphoria is currently the official name of the diagnosis according to the *Diagnostic and Statistical Manual of Mental Disorders, Fifth Edition* (DSM-5).[2] There is debate about whether gender incongruence is a psychiatric diagnosis and whether distress is inherent for the condition. Suffering caused by social stigma, such as family nonacceptance and peer bullying (See Mark L. Hatzenbuehler and John E. Pachankis' article, "Stigma and Minority Stress as Social Determinants of Health among LGBT Youth: Research Evidence and Clinical Implications," in this issue) is fundamentally different from distress caused by gender incongruence itself. A pragmatic improvement in the proposed upcoming eleventh edition of the World Health Organization International Classification of Diseases might be the use of the term "gender incongruence" and the removal from the mental health conditions section.[3]

Increasing numbers of youth with gender incongruence and gender dysphoria are seeking mental health support and medical care. This current increase in interest in gender dysphoria is reflected while searching PubMed on "gender dysphoria"; it shows a sharp increase in the number of publications since the 1970s (**Fig. 1**), especially in the last 2 years (PubMed search, October 19, 2015). When the filter "birth – 18 years" is added, there are 182 hits, with 48 of these publications in 2014 and 2015. However, most articles are opinion or review papers and not original data

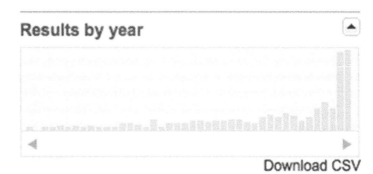

Fig. 1. Number of PubMed hits for gender dysphoria since 1970.

research and hitherto there is only little research evidence for cause, course, and treatment of gender dysphoria.

The existing clinical guidelines of the World Professional Association of Transgender Health and of the Endocrine Society are therefore to a large extent consensus based.[4] This article provides the primary care pediatrician with relevant recent evidence and consensus on childhood and adolescent transgender care and shows how to create a supportive and safe environment for youth with gender incongruence.

PREVALENCE, ETIOLOGIC FACTORS, AND COURSE

Based on the number of referrals to specialized gender identity services, the prevalence rate of gender dysphoria in children and adolescents seems to be low. However, 1% of parents in a large twin study (around 14,000 pairs) endorsed that their prepubertal child "wished to be the opposite sex"[5] and 1.2% of 8000 high school students in another study answered positively when asked "are you transgender" (although 1.7% answered to not understand the question).[6] From these simple questions one cannot infer a gender incongruence diagnosis, so it remains difficult to predict how many youth with gender dysphoria and other gender identity variant youth will seek related medical and mental health care in the near future.

There is some evidence from neuroimaging studies showing that adolescents with gender dysphoria have functional and structural characteristics resembling peers of the experienced gender without gender dysphoria.[7,8] However, other brain functions and structures cannot be distinguished from natal gender control subjects. An important role for genetic factors was revealed by twin studies on gender dysphoria, but there remains a role of the environment explaining around 30% to 38% of the found variance.[5] So at present, biologic, social, and psychological factors are all considered to play a role in gender identity development.

When clinically working with gender identity variant youth it is relevant to make a distinction between prepubertal and postpubertal children (adolescents). The preschool ages between 3 and 7 years are important in normative gender development; around that time most children develop a core sense of being a boy or being a girl according to their assigned gender. They do so while cognitively learning to label gender and grasp the understanding that gender is stable of over time and not dependent on superficial characteristics, such as clothing or behavior.[9]

In various clinic-referred samples of children with gender incongruence who were longitudinally followed into their late adolescent or early adult years, most (85%) were no longer dissatisfied with their birth-assigned gender after puberty; there was an increased likelihood of a homosexual sexual orientation compared with gender-normative developing children.[10] The degree to which these clinical samples are representative of patients seen in general pediatric practice or of the general population is not known. Because the future developmental pathway of these prepubertal children is yet unknown and these children should have the freedom to personally explore their gender identity while growing up, the term gender-fluid or gender-creativity is often used.[11]

In a Dutch qualitative follow-up study from childhood to adolescence with adolescents who were either persisting or desisting in their gender incongruence, they reported that the ages 10 to 13 years seemed crucial for their gender identity development. The experience of physical puberty, the first romantic feelings, and changes in gendered social relationships at that time were considered important. In a quantitative follow-up study from the same clinic, the intensity of gender dysphoria, natal female gender, older age, social transitioning, and cognitive and affective cross-gender identification in childhood were found to be associated with persistence in adolescence in a clinic-referred sample; it is noteworthy that predictors were not entirely similar for natal males and natal females.[12]

Because the chances of desistence are high and changing back to the birth-assigned gender role later is stressful,[10] social gender transition in young children should be carefully considered and benefits and risks be weighted. In contrast to pre-pubertal children, chances of desistence of gender dysphoria are low in clinic-referred adolescents deemed eligible for medical interventions. Therefore, once middle-school age is reached, social transitioning has little chance of regret in clinic-referred samples.

There is now some evidence that gender identity variant youth growing up in a supportive environment can develop into psychologically well-functioning individuals not distinguishable from same-age peers.[13,14] However, other studies show that victimization and discrimination in gender nonconforming youth in general and transgender youth specifically is associated with the tendency to develop emotional and behavioral problems. In the last of three consecutive studies comparing psychological functioning in youth referred to two gender identity clinics, it was concluded that whether reported by parents, by the youth self, or their teachers, poor peer relations was the main predictor of such problems.[15] In a population study, peer victimization fully mediated the association between adolescent gender nonconformity and young adult psychosocial functioning (life satisfaction and depression).[16]

Taking this into account, it is understandable that percentages of anxiety in 21% and depression in 12% to 24% of the adolescent referrals to gender identity clinics are reported.[17,18]

CLINICAL APPROACH

The general practitioner, the primary care pediatrician, or the adolescent medicine specialist may be the first medical professional to whom a child or adolescent with gender dysphoria or other gender identity variance presents. This first encounter is of great importance. Out of shame and fear for stigmatization many transgender adolescents have waited a long time before they seek care. The care provider should therefore be nonjudgmental and respectful. Because the terminology that is used in transgender care is constantly changing and the understanding of the concept of gender is shifting (See Scott E. Hadland and colleagues' article, "Caring for LGBTQ Youth in Inclusive and Affirmative Environments," in this issue), clinicians should be mindful of the adolescent's preferred terminology related to their care. As a billable DSM-5 diagnosis, gender dysphoria may allow access to gender-affirming physical and mental health treatment. However, for those who find this term pathologizing or stigmatizing, it may be preferable to use alternative terms.

In the first contact, the clinician also has the task to identify potential immediate risks and harms before referral to a specialized gender care center.[19] When performing a comprehensive medical and social history, some issues should be specifically addressed: safety at home and at school, substance abuse, and sexual and mental health. If urgent and potential life-threatening problems are present local support and care should be provided to bridge the period before the access of specialized transgender care.

A primary care provider can help to ensure a prepubertal gender identity variant child that specialized medical care (puberty blockers) is not yet necessary and may refer to a mental health professional to cope with stigma and nonacceptance, clarify preferred gender expression, and identity and manage relationships and expectations.

Specialized transgender care, which may consist of medical gender-affirming interventions as illustrated in **Fig. 2**, requires a multidisciplinary approach. For adolescents,

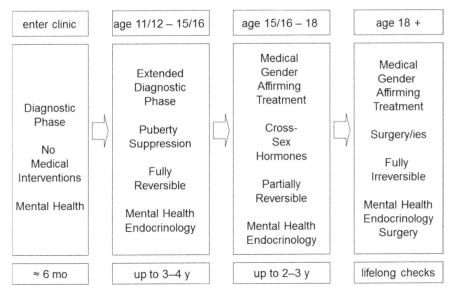

enter clinic	age 11/12 – 15/16	age 15/16 – 18	age 18 +
Diagnostic Phase No Medical Interventions Mental Health	Extended Diagnostic Phase Puberty Suppression Fully Reversible Mental Health Endocrinology	Medical Gender Affirming Treatment Cross-Sex Hormones Partially Reversible Mental Health Endocrinology	Medical Gender Affirming Treatment Surgery/ies Fully Irreversible Mental Health Endocrinology Surgery
≈ 6 mo	up to 3–4 y	up to 2–3 y	lifelong checks

Fig. 2. Multidisciplinary treatment of transgender adolescents.

the core team should consist of mental health professionals (child psychologists, child and adolescent psychiatrists, and other mental health professionals), pediatric medical specialists (endocrinologists, adolescent medicine or other pediatric medical gender specialists), and surgeons (urologists, plastic surgeons, and gynecologists). Also there should be ready access to supporting disciplines when needed, such as dermatologists for permanent hair removal, or pelvic floor physical therapists. The core team ideally meets on a regular basis for team decision making on the steps in care to be taken to support the adolescent with gender dysphoria or other gender identity variance.

Regrettably, these multidisciplinary teams do not exist in every region. A transgender adolescent could then profit from individual caretakers at different locations. Excellent communication between them is a prerequisite.

DIAGNOSIS

The core element of gender dysphoria in the DSM-5 is the incongruence between experienced and assigned gender.[2] There are different indicators of gender dysphoria in children and adolescents/adults. **Boxes 1** and **2** provide a description of the key elements required to make a diagnosis.

Several challenges may complicate the clinical diagnosis of gender dysphoria based on the DSM-5 criteria. Not all children are able to verbalize their thoughts and feelings well. Assessments are usually done by means of (structured) interviews with the parents or other caretakers and the child, and behavioral observations (particularly in young children). School information can also be useful. Besides information on the gender development and current behavior of the child it is also important to obtain a broader picture of child and family functioning.

The diagnostic process for adolescents is similar to what is done in children but more extensive, because in this age group the question is often whether medical interventions are indicated. The recommended procedure in the Standards of Care of the World Professional Association for Transgender Health is a staged one

---

Box 1
DSM-5 key diagnostic elements of a gender dysphoria diagnosis in children

The incongruence between the child's gender identity and the birth-assigned gender is the key criterion of the gender dysphoria diagnosis in children. A strong desire to be the other gender (verbally or nonverbally expressed) is required for a diagnosis. Several other characteristics must be met to be able to make the diagnosis. These characteristics are a preference for cross-dressing, cross-gender roles, and cross-gender interests with regard to play and play-mates. Rejection of gender-typical clothing, gender-typical play, and playmates of the assigned gender are other probable indicators. Aversion against one's physical sex characteristics and a wish for a body typical of the experienced gender may be diagnostic elements, although some prepubescent children might not be concerned about their anatomy. In line with the rationale of the DSM-5, the condition should involve distress or impairment.

(see **Fig. 2**).[4] In the diagnostic phase, the type of gender dysphoria is assessed, and potential factors that may complicate further treatment (eg, adverse social or family circumstances or severe psychopathology) or even lead to posttreatment regret. As a result of the widespread access to the Internet and the increasing public awareness of gender variance, transgender adolescents with nonbinary gender identities became less anxious to disclose these feelings to clinicians. Transgender people (with and without gender identities in-between or outside the female-male spectrum) may not all desire cross-sex hormones (CSH) and gender-affirming surgeries.

TREATMENT
Psychological Interventions

Both for children and adolescents treatment goals may range from dealing with the gender incongruence to focusing on its emotional and social consequences. Psychological interventions may be indicated before (eg, in prepubertal children), during (eg, when adolescents are still rather vulnerable), or even after medical interventions (hormones and surgery).

Young children and their parents often struggle with the question of how to deal with the child's gender incongruence. Parents may not want to deny the child to live according to his/her gender identity, yet may fear negative responses from other people. These families need counseling, information, and support. In case of co-occurring psychopathology or family distress, which may or may not be the result of the gender incongruence, this should be treated. For adolescents, psychotherapy may be helpful to clarify experienced gender identity (eg, when natal boys who were never very feminine in childhood are confused about their desire to cross-dress). Late-onset gender dysphoria (after the start of puberty) leading to hormone treatment and surgery has been described in adolescents[20]; this possibility should be explored in particular.

Box 2
DSM-5 key diagnostic elements of the gender dysphoria diagnosis in adults and adolescents

The incongruence between the adolescents' or adults' gender identity and the birth-assigned gender is the key criterion of the gender dysphoria diagnosis in adults and adolescents. Two diagnostic indicators demonstrating this incongruence should be present to make the diagnosis. Among them are a desire for the anatomy of the experienced gender and an aversion of the body characteristics of the natal sex. Further possible elements involve a desire to be treated as the experienced gender and the feeling that one has the typical emotions and behaviors of the experienced gender. In line with the rationale of the DSM-5, the condition should involve distress or impairment. There is a posttransition specifier to give access to continuing care that supports the new gender assignment.

If adolescents try to adopt other forms of gender expression than male or female (eg "gender queer, or nonbinary" meaning not able to be simply categorized as male or female)[21] they may need support in discovering what suits them best.

If adolescents who seek gender-affirming medical treatment suffer from psychiatric problems these should be treated. Some must be treated before medical treatment starts; others can be taken care of during puberty suppression or gender-affirming hormone therapy preferably by local mental health clinicians.[17,20,22] These local professionals might need the support from transgender specialists with regard to the gender issues or need to seek the proper information from list servers or other Internet resources.

Autism spectrum disorders (ASD) are a special set of psychiatric conditions that may complicate diagnostics and treatment.[23,24] When adolescents with ASD are eligible for medical interventions, including puberty suppression, treatment has to be tailored to the specific ASD problems (eg, procedures have to be explained concretely and long in advance to give the adolescent time to better understand what will happen).

Some families are seriously distressed because of the gender dysphoria and/or medical treatment wish of the adolescent. For instance, parents may have different views about the pace of the transition process of their child or one or more parents/caregivers may not be in support of the diagnosis or treatment. These problems should be addressed early in the course of treatment. Ideally, parents are on board before medical intervention, but there may be cases where the decision is made without one or more caregivers based on the child's needs in accordance with pertinent ethical and legal guidelines related to issues, such as guardianship, status as an emancipated or mature minor, and related issues of informed consent and assent.

If adolescents actually start gender-affirming medical treatment, short- and long-term risks and benefits of medical treatment need to be discussed repeatedly in counseling sessions, because their views, experience, and understanding (eg, of relationships, the impact of infertility, and options for assisted reproductive technologies) change over time (See Sarah M. Wood's article, "HIV, Other Sexually Transmitted Infections, and Sexual and Reproductive Health in LGBT Youth," in this issue). These youth may also need supportive therapy or counseling if the transition is accompanied by adverse or disappointing experiences.

A regular supportive and educational contact with a mental health practitioner during the entire medical gender-affirmative process is often important for an adequate preparation of treatment steps, such as hormones and surgery. Unrealistic transition expectations, such as about changes from hormones or surgery, should be put into perspective. The adolescent also has to be made aware of the importance of a healthy lifestyle early in the diagnostic/treatment process. They should realize that smoking and being overweight creates a higher risk of poor outcomes for hormonal therapy and perioperative and postoperative complications and that, as a consequence, results may cosmetically and functionally be unsatisfactory.

Indications for Puberty Suppression and Cross-Sex Hormones

Young adolescents who have a diagnosis of gender dysphoria and seek medical treatment may be eligible for puberty suppression by means of gonadotrophin-releasing hormone analogues (GnRHa) and CSH. The Standards of Care (seventh edition) of the World Professional Association for Transgender Care give eligibility criteria that have to be fulfilled (**Box 3**).[4]

If puberty-blocking treatment is started around Tanner stages 2 to 3, the very first physical changes are still reversible. Some experience with one's physical puberty is considered valuable because at the onset of puberty it seems to become clear whether

---

Box 3

World Professional Association for Transgender Health gives the following eligibility criteria that have to be fulfilled before any medical treatment is provided (puberty blockers or cross-hormones)

1. The adolescent has demonstrated a long-lasting and intense pattern of gender nonconformity or gender dysphoria (whether suppressed or expressed)

2. Gender dysphoria emerged or worsened with the onset of puberty

3. Any coexisting psychological, medical, or social problems that could interfere with treatment (eg, that may compromise treatment adherence) have been addressed, such that the adolescent's situation and functioning are stable enough to start treatment

4. The adolescent has given informed consent and, particularly when the adolescent has not reached the age of medical consent, the parents or other caretakers or guardians have also given informed consent to the treatment and are involved in supporting the adolescent throughout the treatment process

5. For puberty suppression, the adolescent should further have reached puberty (Tanner stage 2)

Adapted from Coleman E, Bockting W, Botzer M, et al. Standards of care for the health of transsexual, transgender, and gender-nonconforming people, version 7. Int J Transgend 2012;13(4):177; with permission.

---

the gender dysphoria will desist or persist.[10] For CSH, the Endocrine Society guidelines provide an age criterion of 16 years, the first step of actual medical gender-affirming treatment with partially irreversible effects.[25] According to the Dutch approach that was followed in the only long-term evaluative study on puberty suppression followed by gender-affirming treatment, adolescents were considered eligible for puberty suppression at age 12 and for CSH at age 16.[13] At the Dutch clinic where the study was performed, the positive results of the outcome study have led to a more flexible use of the age criteria (see **Fig. 2**). It has yet to be determined, however, how to assess informed consent at young ages and how psychological maturity can be assessed.

Physical Interventions

After the first diagnostic phase during which no medical interventions are provided, endocrine treatment of adolescents with gender dysphoria consists of two phases: the extended diagnostic phase with pubertal suspension or gonadal suppression by means of GnRHa; and the first phase of actual medical gender-affirming treatment with the addition of the sex hormones of the experienced gender (CSH supplementation). Treatment with GnRHa is fully reversible, treatment with CSH only partially (see **Fig. 2**). Surgery is another fully irreversible step of medical gender-affirmative treatment. There is also now increasing flexibility in some care environments about which steps are taken and in what order. For example, some transmales elect to have top surgery first before starting CSH, or choose not to take hormones at all.

Puberty Suppression

GnRHa have been used in the treatment of central precocious puberty since 1981.[26] The use of GnRHa is regarded as safe and effective, with no long-term adverse or irreversible effects.[27] GnRHa can also be used to suspend puberty in adolescents with gender dysphoria and thus prevent the further unwanted development of the natal secondary sex characteristics. GnRHa is generally well tolerated with the exception of hot flushes early in treatment. However, more recently three cases of hypertension under triptorelin treatment were reported. Also, one case was complicated by increased intracranial pressure, which necessitated temporarily cessation of treatment.[28] Increased intracranial pressure is a rare adverse event and usually associated with leuprolide.[29]

Cross-Sex Hormone Therapy

The first actual step of partially irreversible gender-affirming treatment is CSH therapy and generally has two treatment regimes. When GnRHa treatment was started in the early stages of pubertal development, the "new" puberty is induced with a dosage scheme that is also common in hypogonadal patients.[25] Alternatively, when treatment is started long after the start of puberty CSH can be given at a higher start dose and more rapidly increased until maintenance dosage. Under CSH, the secondary sex characteristics of the desired sex develop. For the specific masculinizing and feminizing therapy dosage schemes, see **Fig. 3**.

Surgery

When previous phases have consolidated the diagnosis, and social transition has been satisfactory, the next treatment steps are taken. According to the standards of care of the World Professional Association of Transgender Health: "Genital surgery should not be carried out until patients reach the legal age of majority to give consent for medical procedures in a given country. The age threshold should be seen as a minimum criterion and not an indication in and of itself for active intervention."[4] Depending on what the young adult wants, this phase may consist of various types of surgery. Masculinizing surgeries may include mastectomy or top surgery (if they did not receive early puberty suppression and have significant breast development), hysterectomy/oopherectomy, colpectomy (vaginectomy), and operations on the external genitalia (metaidoioplasty or phalloplasty). Feminizing procedures may include partial penectomy with vaginoplasty and breast augmentation. Transfemales who began puberty suppression at an early age often have insufficient penile skin for a classical vaginoplasty and need an adjusted surgical procedure, such as a technique using colon tissue.

MONITORING AND FOLLOW-UP

So far effects of GnRHa treatment followed by CSH treatment and surgery have been positive,[13,30,31] although evaluation studies largely come from one clinic and confirmation of these results from other clinics is much needed. The promising results, however, do not imply that nobody experiences any problems after treatment. Despite repeated explanations and discussions about what can and cannot be expected of the treatment, certain outcomes (eg, difficulties in finding a partner or undesirable results of surgery) may be disappointing. Of particular interest in this group is the infertility that is associated with treatment before the gonads are fully developed. Although procedures to preserve fertility in prepubertal children are becoming medically possible (eg, cryopreservation of gonadal tissue), they are often not available or expensive for transgender adolescents and future outcome is still unsure. Although parenting was not a major issue when in early adolescence, later in life this may be a different matter and result in grief. Fertility thus should be a focus of counseling (See Sarah M. Wood's article, "HIV, Other Sexually Transmitted Infections, and Sexual and Reproductive Health in LGBT Youth," in this issue).

PHYSICAL CHECK-UPS

Before starting GnRHa a health assessment takes place. It is advised to include in the history the frequency of weight bearing exercise and calcium intake. **Fig. 4** provides further physical examination and additional investigations, also before starting CSH.

From 11–12 y and T2/3	From 15–16 y
Pubertal suspension: GnRHa	**Gender affirming hormones:** Sex steroids

<u>At start</u>

- health assessment
    - Tanner stage
    - BMI
    - blood pressure
- DEXA
    - lumbar spine
    - hip
- metabolic profile
    - liver- and renal function
    - lipids
    - fasting glucose and insulin
- karyotype
    - pre-menarchial girls

<u>At start</u>

- health assessment

- DEXA

- metabolic profile

- side effect screening

    - Masculnizing treatments:
        - hemoglobulin
        - hematocrite

    - Feminizing treatments:
        - prolactin

<u>Follow-up (every 3–6 mo)</u>

- health assessment

- DEXA every 2–3 y

- side effect screening every 1–2 y

Fig. 3. Endocrine treatment in transgender adolescents. Early pubertal transsexual patients are treated with GnRHa to prevent further progression of puberty and thus development of secondary sexual characteristics belonging to their biologic but undesired sex. If the desire for sex reassignment persists, at the age of 16 the sex steroids of the desired sex are added to the GnRHa therapy. Male-to-female transsexual patients are treated with estradiol-17β orally and female-to-male transsexual patients with testosterone by intramuscular injection. Sex reassignment surgery including gonadectomy takes place from the age of 18. The positive psychological effects of this treatment protocol have been clearly demonstrated. BMI, body mass index.

Because the long-term metabolic consequences are still unknown, it is advisable to encourage the adolescent under medical gender-affirmative treatment to adopt a healthy lifestyle with vigilance for excessive weight gain and to refrain from smoking.[25]

CONTROVERSIES

The clinical approach of transgender youth has not been without controversy. In children the debate focuses on whether there should be a gender dysphoria or gender

---

1. Pubertal induction with increasing dosage every six months

Feminizing therapy: 17β-estradiol	Masculinizing therapy: testosterone
• 5 µg/kg/d	• 25 mg/m²/2 wk im.
• 10 µg/kg/d	• 50 mg/m²/2 wk im.
• 15 µg/kg/d	• 75 mg/m²/2 wk im.
• 20 µg/kg/d	• 100 mg/m²/2 wk im.
• max 2 mg/d	

2. When GnRHa started at 15/16 y of age

• Start dosage
  • Feminizing: 1 mg 17β-estradiol /d
  • Masculinizing: 75 mg testosterone/ 2 wk

• After six months
  • Feminizing: 2 mg 17β-estradiol /d
  • Masculinizing: adult dosage

Fig. 4. Sex steroid dosage scheme. Im., intramuscularly.

---

incongruence diagnosis at all in the diagnostic systems (DSM and International Classification of Diseases). Proponents of retaining the child diagnosis consider access to care (needed for proper psychological treatment and reimbursement) as more important than the potential stigma associated with having a child diagnosis. Pathologizing something that is not considered intrinsically pathologic is what concerns opponents. Currently the American Psychological Association decided to leave child and adolescent diagnoses in the DSM-5, but greatly revised their name and criteria to emphasize that dysphoria resulting from gender incongruence, rather than gender incongruence itself or a transgender identity, is the clinical focus. The diagnosis for children has become stricter to prevent diagnosing gender variant behavior only.

Although opinions move in the direction of acceptance, early treatment of young adolescents with gender dysphoria still is a topic of debate.[32] Some fear that a diagnosis of gender dysphoria cannot reliably be made in adolescence, because in this developmental phase gender identity may still be fluctuating. Others fear that puberty suppression will inhibit a spontaneous formation of a consistent gender identity. These fears, however, do not seem to be supported by the studies that have been conducted among adolescents.

There are some safety considerations to be made on the long-term effects because during puberty the bone mass increases and peak bone mass is achieved at the age of 20 to 30. There is now some evidence that under GnRHa treatment bone-mass z scores decreased but after CSH was started, bone mass accrual resumed implying a possible delay in peak bone mass.[33]

In adult transgender health care there are reports on metabolic changes and risk to cardiovascular disease during CSH. So far, there is no evidence that early medical gender-affirmative treatment in adolescence would have a negative effect on cardiovascular health later in life. Long-term follow-up, however, is still necessary to evaluate this risk.

Despite the reservations that existed in the beginning of the treatment approach starting with GnRHa, views on this protocol are rapidly changing.[34] Since 1987, when the first gender identity clinic for children and adolescents, situated first in Utrecht and since 2000 in Amsterdam, was opened in Europe, many other clinics in the world now see children and adolescents with gender dysphoria and use puberty suppression as part of their treatment of adolescents with gender dysphoria.[33–39] However, research on the effects of GnRHa treatment followed by CSH is still scarce, and concerns about long-term effects have to be taken seriously. Results from other centers need to ensure that the treatment is safe (**Box 4**).

Box 4
What is known and what is unknown on gender dysphoria or gender incongruence?

What Is Known	What Is Unknown
Gender incongruent children can show nongender-stereotypical behavior and explicitly insist that they are the other gender at ages as young as 2–3 y.	When gender identity is fixed in gender variant children there is some evidence that the ages between 10 and 13, and the experience of physical puberty is of relevance.
Early longitudinal evidence indicates that early medical interventions (typically older than age 12 y) lead to successful psychological functioning in early adulthood.	Which prepubertal children with gender dysphoria will be adolescents/adults with gender dysphoria.
Early longitudinal evidence on bone development suggests some potential reduction in bone mass in young adulthood as a consequence of puberty suppression earlier.	Long-term psychological and physical outcome into later adulthood of adolescents treated with puberty suppression.
Early studies indicate that puberty suppression has no negative influence on an executive functioning task indicative of healthy pubertal brain development.	Outcomes of child and adolescent transgender care including puberty suppression of non-Dutch and non-European gender identity clinics.
Early brain imaging studies suggest that transgender adolescents have certain brain morphology and brain functioning in the direction of their experienced gender.	

SUMMARY

The recognition and acknowledgment of gender incongruence and gender dysphoria in children and adolescents has evolved impressively over the last two decades. Not long ago youth and parents were hardly aware that children and adolescents could experience gender dysphoria. Media attention and the Internet have informed society in this respect and have also led to more acceptance and destigmatization of youth with gender dysphoria and transgender youth. In parallel, transgender care for children and adolescents has developed and is now much more widely available. Controversies and many challenges continue to exist, however, around clinical management of gender variant children and adolescents. Most clinical guidelines are consensus based and research evidence is limited. Clinicians should therefore be humble and careful in the advice and treatments that they provide and open with patients and families about this lack of evidence. The introduction of puberty suppression as part of clinical management has made medical intervention at a young age possible and has become a valuable element of adolescent transgender care. However, long-term evidence for its success comes only from one clinic, and the ages that puberty suppression and CSH were started in those studies were 12 years and 16 years, respectively. These uncertainties should be weighed against the risk of harming a transgender adolescent when medical intervention is denied.

REFERENCES

1. Adelson SL, American Academy of Child and Adolescent Psychiatry (AACAP) Committee on Quality Issues (CQI). Practice parameter on gay, lesbian, or bisexual sexual orientation, gender nonconformity, and gender discordance in children and adolescents. J Am Acad Child Adolesc Psychiatry 2012;51(9): 957–74.
2. American Psychiatric Association. Diagnostic and statistical manual of mental disorders. 5th edition. Washington, DC: American Psychiatric Publishing; 2013.
3. Drescher J, Cohen-Kettenis P, Winter S. Minding the body: situating gender identity diagnoses in the ICD-11. Int Rev Psychiatry 2012;24(6):568–77.
4. Coleman E, Bockting W, Botzer M, et al. Standards of care for the health of transsexual, transgender, and gender-nonconforming people, version 7. Int J Transgend 2012;13(4):165–232.
5. van Beijsterveldt CE, Hudziak JJ, Boomsma DI. Genetic and environmental influences on cross-gender behavior and relation to behavior problems: a study of Dutch twins at ages 7 and 10 years. Arch Sex Behav 2006;35(6):647–58.
6. Clark TC, Lucassen MF, Bullen P, et al. The health and well-being of transgender high school students: results from the New Zealand adolescent health survey (Youth'12). J Adolesc Health 2014;55(1):93–9.
7. Burke SM, Cohen-Kettenis PT, Veltman DJ, et al. Hypothalamic response to the chemo-signal androstadienone in gender dysphoric children and adolescents. Front Endocrinol 2014;5:60.
8. Hoekzema E, Schagen SE, Kreukels BP, et al. Regional volumes and spatial volumetric distribution of gray matter in the gender dysphoric brain. Psychoneuroendocrinology 2015;55:59–71.
9. Ruble DN, Martin CL, Berenbaum SA. Gender development. In: Eisenberg N, Damon W, Lerner RM, editors. Handbook of child psychology: vol. 3, Social, emotional, and personality development. 6th edition. Hoboken (NJ): John Wiley & Sons Inc; 2006. p. 858–932.

10. Steensma TD, Biemond R, Boer FD, et al. Desisting and persisting gender dysphoria after childhood: a qualitative follow-up study. Clin Child Psychol Psychiatry 2011;16(4):499–516.

11. Ehrensaft D. From gender identity disorder to gender identity creativity: true gender self child therapy. J Homosex 2012;59(3):337–56.

12. Steensma TD, McGuire JK, Kreukels BP, et al. Factors associated with desistence and persistence of childhood gender dysphoria: a quantitative follow-up study. J Am Acad Child Adolesc Psychiatry 2013;52(6):582–90.

13. de Vries AL, McGuire JK, Steensma TD, et al. Young adult psychological outcome after puberty suppression and gender reassignment. Pediatrics 2014;134(4): 696–704.

14. Olson KR, Durwood L, DeMeules M, et al. Mental health of transgender children who are supported in their identities. Pediatrics 2016;137(3):1–8.

15. de Vries AL, Steensma TD, Cohen-Kettenis PT, et al. Poor peer relations predict parent- and self-reported behavioral and emotional problems of adolescents with gender dysphoria: a cross-national, cross-clinic comparative analysis. Eur Child Adolesc Psychiatry 2016;25(6):579–88.

16. Toomey RB, Ryan C, Diaz RM, et al. Gender-nonconforming lesbian, gay, bisexual, and transgender youth: school victimization and young adult psychosocial adjustment. Dev Psychol 2010;46(6):1580–9.

17. de Vries AL, Doreleijers TA, Steensma TD, et al. Psychiatric comorbidity in gender dysphoric adolescents. J Child Psychol Psychiatry 2011;52(11):1195–202.

18. Olson J, Schrager SM, Belzer M, et al. Baseline physiologic and psychosocial characteristics of transgender youth seeking care for gender dysphoria. J Adolesc Health 2015;57(4):374–80.

19. Guss C, Shumer D, Katz-Wise SL. Transgender and gender nonconforming adolescent care: psychosocial and medical considerations. Curr Opin Pediatr 2015;27(4):421–6.

20. Zucker KJ, Bradley SJ, Owen-Anderson A, et al. Demographics, behavior problems, and psychosexual characteristics of adolescents with gender identity disorder or transvestic fetishism. J Sex Marital Ther 2012;38(2):151–89.

21. Janssen A, Erickson-Schroth L. A new generation of gender: learning patience from our gender nonconforming patients. J Am Acad Child Adolesc Psychiatry 2013;52(10):995–7.

22. Skagerberg E, Davidson S, Carmichael P. Internalizing and externalizing behaviors in a group of young people with gender dysphoria. Int J Transgend 2013; 14(3):105–12.

23. de Vries AL, Noens IL, Cohen-Kettenis PT, et al. Autism spectrum disorders in gender dysphoric children and adolescents. J Autism Dev Disord 2010;40(8): 930–6.

24. Van Der Miesen AI, Hurley H, De Vries AL. Gender dysphoria and autism spectrum disorder: a narrative review. Int Rev Psychiatry 2016;28(1):70–80.

25. Hembree WC, Cohen-Kettenis P, Delemarre-van de Waal HA, et al. Endocrine treatment of transsexual persons: an Endocrine Society clinical practice guideline. J Clin Endocrinol Metab 2009;94(9):3132–54.

26. Laron Z, Kauli R, Zeev ZB, et al. D-TRP5-analogue of luteinizing hormone releasing hormone in combination with cyproterone acetate to treat precocious puberty. Lancet 1981;2(8253):955–6.

27. Carel JC, Eugster EA, Rogol A, et al. Consensus statement on the use of gonadotropin-releasing hormone analogs in children. Pediatrics 2009;123(4): e752–62.

28. Klink D, Bokenkamp A, Dekker C, et al. Arterial Hypertension as a Complication of Triptorelin Treatment in Adolescents with Gender Dysphoria. Endocrinol Metab Int J 2015;2(1).
29. Arber N, Shirin H, Fadila R, et al. Pseudotumor cerebri associated with leuprorelin acetate. Lancet 1990;335(8690):668.
30. de Vries AL, Steensma TD, Doreleijers TA, et al. Puberty suppression in adolescents with gender identity disorder: a prospective follow-up study. J Sex Med 2011;8(8):2276–83.
31. Cohen-Kettenis PT, Schagen SE, Steensma TD, et al. Puberty suppression in a gender-dysphoric adolescent: a 22-year follow-up. Arch Sex Behav 2011;40(4):843–7.
32. Korte A, Lehmkuhl U, Goecker D, et al. Gender identity disorders in childhood and adolescence: currently debated concepts and treatment strategies. Dtsch Arztebl Int 2008;105(48):834–41.
33. Klink D, Caris M, Heijboer A, et al. Bone mass in young adulthood following gonadotropin-releasing hormone analog treatment and cross-sex hormone treatment in adolescents with gender dysphoria. J Clin Endocrinol Metab 2015;100(2):E270–5.
34. Cohen-Kettenis PT, Delemarre-van de Waal HA, Gooren LJ. The treatment of adolescent transsexuals: changing insights. J Sex Med 2008;5(8):1892–7.
35. Hsieh S, Leininger J. Resource list: clinical care programs for gender-nonconforming children and adolescents. Pediatr Ann 2014;43(6):238–44.
36. Hewitt JK, Paul C, Kasiannan P, et al. Hormone treatment of gender identity disorder in a cohort of children and adolescents. Med J Aust 2012;196(9):578–81.
37. Khatchadourian K, Amed S, Metzger DL. Clinical management of youth with gender dysphoria in Vancouver. J Pediatr 2014;164(4):906–11.
38. Nakatsuka M. Adolescents with gender identity disorder: reconsideration of the age limits for endocrine treatment and surgery. Seishin Shinkeigaku Zasshi 2012;114(6):647–53 [in Japanese].
39. Fisher AD, Ristori J, Bandini E, et al. Medical treatment in gender dysphoric adolescents endorsed by SIAMS-SIE-SIEDP-ONIG. J Endocrinol Invest 2014;37(7):675–87.

National Resources for Lesbian, Gay, Bisexual, Transgender Youth, Providers, and Support Persons

In caring for LGBT youth, pediatric practitioners may find a number of community resources helpful for addressing the needs that are discussed throughout this volume. These may be found at local, state, national, and international levels. As an example and a partial resource list, below are some national/international organizations. The list is neither exhaustive nor definitive, but may be useful for practitioners to consider and use to further explore options. It includes information about these organizations' services.

FOR PROVIDERS

American Academy of Child and Adolescent Psychiatry (www.aacap.org)

The American Academy of Child and Adolescent Psychiatry provides several mental health resources relevant to lesbian, gay, bisexual, transgender (LGBT) youth and families, including best-practice guidelines (Practice Parameters), patient education materials (Facts for Families), and other guidelines and resources.

American Academy of Pediatrics Section on Lesbian, Gay, Bisexual, Transgender Health and Wellness (www.aap.org)

The SOLGBTHW of the American Academy of Pediatrics is a group of pediatricians and other health providers interested in LGBT health and wellness.

American Psychiatric Association (www.psychiatry.org)

The American Psychiatric Association provides mental health resources relevant to LGBT patients, including youth and families, including practice guidelines and position papers, a best-practice highlights guideline called "Working with LGBTQ Patients," and a Gay, Lesbian and Bisexual Caucus for practitioners.

Gay and Lesbian Medical Association (www.glma.org)

The Gay and Lesbian Medical Association (GLMA) is an international organization of LGBT health care professionals and their supporters that focuses on ensuring health care equality for LGBT individuals. Members of GLMA use their individual expertise to address the health and well-being of LGBT people, specifically through health care reform, continuing education of health care professionals, and hospital discrimination. The Web site provides a directory of providers with competence in LGBT health care.

National Lesbian, Gay, Bisexual, Transgender Health Education Center (www. lgbthealtheducation.org)

The National LGBT Health Education Center focuses on providing resources and educational programs to health care organizations and providers to optimize care for LGBT people.

Pediatr Clin N Am 63 (2016) 1137–1139
http://dx.doi.org/10.1016/j.pcl.2016.09.001
0031-3955/16

World Professional Association for Transgender Health (www.wpath.org)

The World Professional Association for Transgender Health (WPATH) is a professional organization dedicated to providing high-quality health care for transgender, transsexual, and gender-nonconforming individuals. The organization connects professionals across a variety of fields to further the understanding and treatment of gender identity disorder. The Web site provides a directory of providers with competence in transgender health care.

FOR YOUTH AND FAMILIES
Advocates for Youth (www.advocatesforyouth.org)

Advocates for Youth partners with youth leaders, adult allies, and youth-serving organizations to advocate for policies and champion programs that recognize young people's rights to honest sexual health information; accessible, confidential, and affordable sexual health services; and the resources and opportunities necessary to create sexual health equity for all youth.

Crisis Text Line (www.crisistextline.org/textline/)

Crisis Text Line is a free, national, 24-hour text line that provides counseling for people in any type of crisis.

Family Acceptance Project (http://familyproject.sfsu.edu)

The Family Acceptance Project (FAP) is a research, intervention, education, and policy initiative designed to decrease the risks faced by LGBT youth (homelessness, human immunodeficiency virus, suicide) by promoting family support and well-being. The initiative focuses on the impact families can have on the risk and well-being of their LGBT children, and provides training on their family interventional approach to providers, families, and religious leaders worldwide.

Gay Lesbian & Straight Education Network (www.glsen.org)

The Gay Lesbian & Straight Education Network (GLSEN) is an organization that seeks to end discrimination, harassment, and bullying caused by sexual identity, gender identity, and gender expression in K-12 schools. GLSEN provides educational resources for educators, advocates for inclusive safe school policies, and conducts research to inform legislators of the issues LGBT youth face, as well as developing best practices and resources to create a safe school environment.

Parents, Families, Friends, and Allies United with Lesbian, Gay, Bisexual, Transgender People (www.pflag.org)

Parents, Families, Friends, and Allies United with LGBT People (PFLAG) is the nation's largest nonprofit organization for LGBT allies and family, with more than 500 chapters across the country. PFLAG focuses on providing support for LGBT families, educating the broader public on issues faced by members of the LGBT community, and advocating for policies and laws that promote LGBT equality.

stopbullying.gov (www.stopbullying.gov)

This is a Web site run by the US Department of Health and Human Services that provides information on bullying, cyberbullying, people at risk, and how to prevent and respond to bullying.

Substance Abuse and Mental Health Services Administration National Suicide Resources (www.suicidepreventionlifeline.org)

The National Suicide Prevention Lifeline is a toll-free, confidential suicide prevention hotline available 24-hours a day. Crisis counseling and mental health referrals are regularly provided: 1-800-273-TALK.

The Trevor Project (www.thetrevorproject.org/pages/get-help-now#tc)

The Trevor Project is a nonprofit organization that focuses on crisis intervention and suicide prevention for LGBT youth. It provides free and confidential phone, instant message, and text messaging crisis intervention services through the Trevor Lifeline (866-488-7386), TrevorChat, and TrevorText. TrevorSpace also provides a safe and secure social networking site that connects LGBT youth around the world.

True Colors Fund (www.truecolorsfund.org)

The True Colors Fund is a philanthropic organization that aims to end homelessness among LGBT youth by educating the public and advocating within government agencies.

Index

Note: Page numbers of article titles are in **boldface** type.

Pediatr Clin N Am 63 (2016) 1141–1150
http://dx.doi.org/10.1016/S0031-3955(16)41122-3
0031-3955/16

Moving?

Make sure your subscription moves with you!

To notify us of your new address, find your **Clinics Account Number** (located on your mailing label above your name), and contact customer service at:

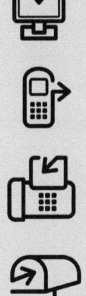

Email: journalscustomerservice-usa@elsevier.com

800-654-2452 (subscribers in the U.S. & Canada)
314-447-8871 (subscribers outside of the U.S. & Canada)

Fax number: 314-447-8029

Elsevier Health Sciences Division
Subscription Customer Service
3251 Riverport Lane
Maryland Heights, MO 63043

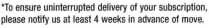

*To ensure uninterrupted delivery of your subscription, please notify us at least 4 weeks in advance of move.

Printed and bound by CPI Group (UK) Ltd, Croydon, CR0 4YY

03/10/2024

01040393-0002